THE ARTHRITIS CODE

DAVID ROBIN

Copyright © 2020 David Robin

All rights reserved.

DEDICATION

To my wife, Helen, and my daughter, Susan.

CONTENTS

Introduction	1
Chapter 1: The Causes of Arthritis	3
Chapter 2: The Types of Arthritis	9
Chapter 3: What Is the Gerson Method?	15
Chapter 4: Restoring Health	19
Chapter 5: Making Your Home Gerson Friendly	27
Chapter 6: Choosing the Right Foods	35
Chapter 7: Enemas for the Gerson Method	51
Chapter 8: What You Need to Know about Medication	59
Chapter 9: Healing Reactions	67
Chapter 10: Avoiding Pitfalls When Using the Gerson Method	73
Chapter 11: Your Questions Answered	79
Chapter 12: Dealing with Stress	85
Chapter 13: What to Expect After the Gerson Method	89
Chapter 14: Further Resources	93
Conclusion	95

INTRODUCTION

If you have arthritis, then you know how debilitating the condition is. It can keep you from doing anything you enjoy. More than that, it can hinder your everyday life too.

People develop arthritis fairly commonly, so we often just assume it is a part of life. We associate it with aging or autoimmune diseases. We shrug it off and then just try to get by, taking medications that only cause more problems.

What if there was a way to overcome arthritis, and we aren't just talking about finding relief for a day or two. We are talking about the question: what if you could be free of arthritis for the rest of your life?

That question is not absurd no matter what you have been told over and over again by traditional doctors. In fact, there is a solution to your problems, and it comes in the form of the Gerson Method.

Right now, you have a lot of things going wrong in your body, and all of those things culminate, for you, in the form of arthritis. Other people experience other things, even serious conditions like heart disease and cancer. What you don't realize though is that the things going wrong in your body can be fixed.

There are two reasons why people develop illness:

- Lack of nutrients
- High levels of toxins

We are going to discuss what that means in more detail later, but what you must keep in mind right now is that there is relief available. You actually have the ability to completely heal from arthritis, and everything you need to do that comes in the form of your own body.

You don't need medications. You don't need chemicals.

All you need is within you. Your body is a powerful tool, and right now, it is being held back from healing itself.

The Gerson Method is the answer for you, and through this book, you will learn everything you need to know about this therapy. If you are ready to embark on a journey that will bring total health and wellness to your body, then read on. What you need to know is right here, and the tools you need to heal are right within yourself.

It's time to make a change in your life, and that change has nothing to do with going to the right doctor or finding the right prescription medication. What it does have to do with is your own body and its ability to heal itself. So, start learning right now and you can see how the Gerson Method is right for you.

CHAPTER 1: THE CAUSES OF ARTHRITIS

Before you can really understand how to cure your arthritis, you need to know what caused it in the first place. After all, knowing the cause can lead directly to the cure. If you spend time reading medical texts and you do research online, you will run into the same thing over and over again: people, doctors, and researchers all have theories on why arthritis develops, but no one really knows what the actual cause is.

So, instead of taking traditional paths to treat conditions, which usually involve just taking medications to cover up symptoms, the Gerson Method looks at things very differently. That take on the condition has to do with actually finding the root cause, which is almost always linked to nutrition.

This book is designed to educate you on curing your illness with the Gerson Method, and so the causes of arthritis included here are based on this method, as well.

Look at Your Own Body

I want you to take a look at yourself. I mean, really look at yourself, including your teeth. They aren't made to eat animal products. If you consider the teeth of a true carnivore, like a cat, you will notice that they are very sharp and pointed. That's because they are used to tear into animal meat. Your own teeth, however, are blunt. Do you know what that means? They are made for eating vegetables, not animals.

Then, there is your stomach. The acids in your stomach are weak compared to carnivorous animals. Animals like dogs and cats have enough stomach acid to break down meat and even bone. Your stomach does not. Again, this is another sign you aren't meant to be eating animal products.

What does it have to do with arthritis? Animal products don't break down properly in our digestive system, and as a result, they leave toxins behind. A good example of this is milk. There have been documented cases of people developing arthritis soon after they began consuming large amounts of milk. We are always taught that dairy products are good for us, so we add them to our diet in massive amounts. We attempt to ensure our teeth and bones are healthy by drinking milk by the glassful, but what we don't realize is that we are actually poisoning our bodies.

In fact, milk is such a common culprit that even medical doctors who aren't sure what causes arthritis have indicated that anyone who already has rheumatoid arthritis should avoid dairy.

> *"RA symptoms may flare as a response to specific proteins found in dairy products. Some people with rheumatoid arthritis who report intolerance to milk have antibodies to milk proteins. The body forms these antibodies to protect itself from what it mistakenly perceives as a harmful substance." (Lio, n.d.)*

Do you think your body would create antibodies for no reason? Not at all! And, the fact that a human body would create an antibody because of milk tells you right there that dairy doesn't belong in your system.

That's only the beginning, too. You may already know that cattle are given antibiotics and other medications to remain healthy while being used to provide milk. Those medications find their way into the milk itself and then you consume them. It's sort of like consuming poison.

Your Metabolism

Your body and all of its processes run on something called the metabolism. As you probably already know, your metabolism will have an impact on how easily you can lose or gain weight.

People who are overweight tend to have a slower metabolism while people who are thinner tend to have a faster metabolism. However, weight is not the only thing affected by this process within your body.

A disturbed or disrupted metabolism can have a massive impact on whether or not you develop arthritis. And, there are numerous things that can cause this disruption:

- Animal Proteins – We are told over and over again that we need these proteins to be healthy, but they are not processed and metabolized in the body properly. They aren't meant for us and they cause more harm than good.
- Food Processes – It seems we are always finding ways to process foods and make them simply not good for us. Deep-frying foods ruins their healthily qualities. Adding additives to keep foods good for a longer time or to make them more tasteful are other ways we change foods to the point that they actually disrupt our metabolism.
- Chemicals – The foods that actually will make you healthy – the ones that come from the earth – are ruined by chemicals and pesticides. When these things are used on plants and vegetables, the foods themselves become saturated, and that means you consume pesticides and all sorts of chemicals that work as toxins in the body.
- Salt – We tend to add salt to everything, as a flavor additive and as a way to preserve foods. However, salt is extremely bad for the body, causing it to retain water and to work as a toxin in the system. Salt is toxic for the tissue, the kidneys, and the digestive system.
- Medications – When your metabolism is disturbed and you go to the doctor, they will prescribe medications for any pain you are experiencing. However, those medications do not cure the condition. They actually just make it worse.
- Outside Toxins – In addition to toxins that may be added to your food sources, there are toxins in the very air around you, and they can all work to disturb your metabolism and make arthritis worse. Some of these toxins include car exhaust, factory waste, cleaning chemicals, chemicals added to drinking water, and more.
- Deficiencies – The foods you are eating are deficient in what your body needs, like collagen, and this means you are deficient, too. Processed foods don't have the vitamins, minerals, and enzymes your body needs, and as a result, you

are consuming empty calories that will not help you at all. When your body is deficient, it will begin to fight back in an attempt to right itself. As a result, certain types of arthritis will develop.

- The Problem of New Science – Scientists and researchers are always looking for something new and unique to offer, and often that comes in the form of "New Science" that actually does more harm than good. After all, we already know that vaccines that are meant to keep children well have actually made them sick, and vaccines have even been associated with autism. So many things that have been attributed to "New Science" have actually made people unwell.

So, what actually causes arthritis? If you read articles written by doctors and scientists, they will usually point to a few things. In fact, the Mayo Clinic states that osteoarthritis simply is a "fact of life" due to wear and tear on joints. It goes on to state that rheumatoid arthritis is an autoimmune condition, which would imply the body is attacking itself. (Causes, n.d.)

That train of thought simply doesn't make sense though. The body is made to function properly for the extent of our lives. Why would it attack itself? Why would it begin wearing out? These common "causes" aren't actually the causes at all. Instead, it is eating the wrong foods, being exposed to toxins, and taking the wrong approach to treatment.

Every day, right now, you are exposed to things that actually form the cause. You come in contact with chemicals and toxins. You eat animal products. You drink milk. All of these things have a negative impact on your body and can seriously disturb your metabolism. Then, you go to the doctor and you are prescribed medication – which only masks the symptoms and can cause serious damage to the body. You don't get a cure. You get a "cover" and it doesn't do anything to help you.

The key to understanding the Gerson Method and actually curing your condition comes in the form of pinpointing the cause. Once you have done that, as discussed in this chapter, you will be able to begin pursuing your treatment. It is actually very possible to cure arthritis despite what you may have been told by doctors, and the cure doesn't come in the form you may expect.

In the next chapter, we will discuss the actual types of arthritis so that you can get a better understanding of what you have wrong with your body, not what a doctor may have said you have wrong. After that, we will go into detail about how the Gerson Method works and how it can be used to cure your own arthritis.

CHAPTER 2: THE TYPES OF ARTHRITIS

What many people don't understand is that there are actually many different types of arthritis. Each of them does have similar symptoms, but are different in their causes, as well.

The Gerson Method can help you overcome any type of the condition, but having a better understanding arthritis is the best way to understand what is going on with your body, so before we delve fully into the Method itself and how to use it, let's take a moment to discuss the types of arthritis from which you could suffer.

Osteoarthritis

Many people consider osteoarthritis as the wear and tear type, meaning that it develops from wear and tear on joints over time.

However, as we have already mentioned in the first chapter of this book, arthritis doesn't just develop for no reason whatsoever. It has to do with foods you eat and environmental factors you are exposed to.

However, what you should note is that osteoarthritis is considered the most common type and it occurs in certain joints, including the hips, spine, knees, neck, toes, and fingers. Often, people experience osteoarthritis in joints that have been previously injured.

When osteoarthritis becomes a problem, the joint itself loses flexibility and it becomes painful and swollen. It may worsen and lessen from time to time. (Osteoarthritis Health Center, n.d.)

Rheumatoid Arthritis

Instead of affecting the cushioning between the joints, as with osteoarthritis, rheumatoid arthritis actually affects the lining around the joint itself.

This leads to swelling, pain, and even deformation. If the condition is not treated, then it can lead to erosion of the bone and loss of use of the hands, where it appears the most.

Rheumatoid arthritis is considered an autoimmune condition, which in medical terms, means that the body attacks itself. Again, this simply doesn't make sense based on how the human body works, and would only imply that an outside source would result in the condition. (Rheumatoid Arthritis, n.d.)

Lupus

The name lupus is not one condition, but a whole group of illnesses, also referred to as autoimmune diseases. There are various symptoms of lupus that can affect the entire body, leading to such problems as:

- Arthritis in the wrists, hands, knees, ankles, and elbows. This includes swelling and aching in those joints.
- Kidney problems that lead to swelling in the hands and feet and water retention.
- Low-grade fever that comes and goes.
- Fatigue that is either extreme and excessive or that lasts for a very long time.
- Rashes and skin problems that appear on the hands, neck, face, back, and arms.
- Rash that creates a butterfly shape across the cheeks and nose.
- Shortness of breath or chest pain when attempting to breathe deeply.
- Sensitivity to the sunlight.
- Alopecia (hair loss)
- Re-occurrence of seizures.
- Easy tendency toward bruising.
- Development of anxiety, memory loss, and depression.

- Problems with blood clotting properly.
- A condition called Raynaud's phenomenon, which means the fingers turn red, blue, or white when exposed to cold.
- Unexplained weight loss or weight gain.
- Ulcers that develop in the mouth and nose.

Even medical doctors who believe autoimmune conditions exist understand that lupus often develops from outside sources, including chemical exposure from smoking, medications, and compounds in drinking water.

One of the most commonly exhibited symptoms of lupus is arthritis in the small joints. (What Is Lupus?, n.d.)

Mixed Collagen Disease

Also referred to as mixed connective tissue disease, this is another condition referred to as autoimmune in nature.

Connective tissues are the things that connect parts of the body together, including muscles, tendons, joints, and bones.

Collagen is the main type of connective tissue, and another one is elastin. There are different types of mixed collagen diseases, including:

- Marfan syndrome, which leads to problems with the connective tissues in the eyes, skeletal system, heart, and lungs.
- Ehlers-Danlos syndrome, which leads to loose skin as well as joints that easily hyperextend.
- Pseudoxanthoma elasticum is a condition that affects elastin specifically.

All of these diseases produce symptoms of polymyositis, rheumatoid arthritis, and systematic lupus.

Again, since this is classified as an auto immune condition, but since we do not believe autoimmune conditions exist, we know that outside factors and toxins lead to this disease as well. (Mixed Connective Tissue Disease (MCTD), n.d.)

Scleroderma

Also referred to as systematic sclerosis, this is also classified as an autoimmune disease. The symptoms of scleroderma actually vary between visible and invisible symptoms. They include:

- One of the outward symptoms is the hardening of patches of skin. This results in tight, swollen, and inflamed areas that can restrict movement.
- Many people with scleroderma will experience numbness, color change, and pain in the fingers and toes whenever they are exposed to cold.
- The condition also can attack the joints, especially in the extremities, causing arthritis.
- Another internal symptom of scleroderma is acid reflux, slow or sluggish intestines, and other digestive upset.
- In some of the most severe cases of scleroderma, the condition has led to serious function problems in the organs such as kidneys, heart, and lungs.

Again, doctors point to the body turning on itself as the case of scleroderma, indicating that an overactive immune system leads to the condition.

However, again, we believe that there has to be something on the outside that is causing the problem in the body and we know that it is food, chemicals, and other environmental factors. (What Is Scleroderma, n.d.)

Ankylosing Spondylitis

This is a condition that specifically affects the back and vertebrae, but it can spread to the ribs, as well.

In this case, it will cause inflammation to the point that some of the vertebrae can actually fuse together, causing back pain and loss of motion.

Additionally, if ankylosing spondylitis does spread to the ribs, this can make it difficult for the person to take deep breaths. Occasionally, the condition can develop in other parts of the body, including the eyes, pelvis, and shoulders. (Ankylosing Spondylitis, n.d.)

Gout

Gout can actually affect different joints in the body, but most commonly, it is found in the big toe. When gout attacks, it causes severe pain, swelling, redness, and tenderness around the joint area.

Gout is considered a form of arthritis, but is very complex due to its nature. The actual medical cause of gout is a buildup of urate crystals within the joint as uric acid builds up in the bloodstream.

When too much uric acid does built up in the blood stream, it can allow the crystals to settle in different joints.

Again, outside factors do cause this buildup and can have a direct effect on whether or not a person will develop gout. (Gout, n.d.)

Fibromyalgia

For many years, people didn't quite understand fibromyalgia as a real condition. That's because it has widespread conditions throughout the body. Essentially, it has an impact on how the brain processes pain and can actually make pain feel much worse. Symptoms of fibromyalgia include:

- Pain throughout the body, including a dull ache that never goes away. Sometimes, it occurs above the waist on both sides of the body.
- Regular fatigue, since the condition causes regular pain. Many people develop sleep disorders including sleep apnea and restless leg syndrome.
- A condition that impairs cognitive ability, which is often referred to as "fibro fog." People may find it very hard to focus on the task at hand, pay attention to things around them, or concentrate on what they need to be doing.

These are not the only symptoms of fibromyalgia either. It can also cause pain and swelling in the joints, depression from the chronic pain, headaches, and abdominal cramps. (Fibromyalgia Symptoms, n.d.)

Osteoporosis

Osteoporosis is a bone disease commonly associated with older women. It develops as the bones become thinner and more brittle.

The condition can weaken the bones to the point that even a single stumble and fall can lead to a broken bone or two. Commonly, osteoporosis affects the back, hips, and wrists.

Doctors will indicate that osteoporosis is a product of age and lack of calcium in the bones, but that is not the case. Here are some important facts that you may not know:

- A study performed at Harvard University found that not only does drinking milk do nothing to help prevent osteoporosis, but that milk can actually cause the disease. People who consumed fewer dairy products were less likely to develop osteoporosis.
- The Yale University School of Medicine has an ongoing study that links osteoporosis directly with the consumption of animal proteins. Additionally, a study in China backs this up, stating that consumption of animal proteins actually causes the bones to dissolve.
- The acid and other chemicals in sodas have been linked to osteoporosis in a study performed by Tufts University.

So, what does this tell you? When you consume foods your body cannot use and when you are exposed to chemicals, you are at a much higher chance of developing this condition. It is absolutely not a byproduct of age. (Snyder, 2012)

There are many different conditions that cause arthritis in one form or another, and unfortunately, these two conditions are most commonly associated with autoimmune illness.

The very idea of autoimmune conditions would imply that the body just randomly attacks itself.

However, the body would have no reason to do this except for the introduction of chemicals and products that our body can't use and products that act as a poison to the body, as well.

So, now that we have gone over what may be wrong with you, it's time to offer the solution, and it comes in the form of the Gerson Method. That's what we will discuss in the next chapter.

CHAPTER 3: WHAT IS THE GERSON METHOD?

Dating back to the 1930s, the Gerson Therapy Method has been providing relief to people with arthritis as well as other conditions including tuberculosis, cancer, and diabetes. The very idea of this therapy is that it uses the body's own power to heal itself by removing toxins and ensuring it is getting the nutrients it needs.

This whole method was developed by Dr. Max Gerson, who stumbled on the ability of his methods after treating a patient with a diet made specially to fend off migraines. The same patient had skin tuberculosis, and their symptoms eased when they were on this diet. When this was discovered, Gerson began researching the diet in more detail.

Dr. Max Gerson

Born in 1881 in Wongrowitz, Germany, Dr. Gerson attended school at Wuerzburg in Berlin as well as in Freiburg. After he discovered that his migraine diet could actually cure skin tuberculosis, his treatments became so popular that the Munich University Hospital allowed him to use their facilities to perform a clinical trial. Out of the 450 patients treated, a total of 446 of those patients fully recovered from their condition.

In 1938, Dr. Gerson came to the United States and passed his board exams to practice medicine in New York. Soon, he was able to make a presentation showing healed cancer patients to the board at the Pepper-Neely Congressional Subcommittee.

Through his clinical trials and his work, Gerson published many different papers and books to show how his method has been extremely helpful at curing many types of illnesses. (Dr. Max Gerson, n.d.)

Charlotte Gerson

After Dr. Gerson passed away in 1959, his daughter, Charlotte, began continuing his work with the Gerson Method. She promoted the therapy and was able to eventually found the Gerson Institute in 1977. Located in San Diego, California, this institute continues to focus on the treatment of a variety of different diseases, including cancer and arthritis.

In addition to the institute in California, there are two licensed clinics that employ the Gerson Method. These include:

- The Gerson Clinic in Mexico – This licensed clinic allows patients to visit and stay for at least two weeks (three weeks is considered optimum) to receive treatment and therapy for a variety of different conditions. The clinic is all-inclusive, which means patients can pay one fee to cover their treatment, boarding, and meals for the entire stay.
- The Gerson Health Centre in Hungary – This licensed clinic began operation in 2009. This center, located outside of Budapest, offers two week sessions for the treatment of a variety of different conditions. Again, when a patient pays, the cost will cover their stay, their treatment, and their meals. Sessions at this location do follow a schedule, however, so patients would need to sign up for a session specifically.

All of the therapies offered at these locations and through the Gerson Method focus on ridding the body of toxins, as well as rectifying any nutritional deficiencies by ensuring the right foods are consumed and that all toxins and chemicals are avoided.

Gerson Therapy for More than Arthritis

While the focus of this book is arthritis, it is very important to discuss the fact that the Gerson Method can be used for a variety of different conditions, and has proven again and again to be extremely successful. These conditions include:

- Cancers (breast cancer, prostate cancer, pancreatic cancer, colon cancer, lymphoma, melanoma and more.)
- Diabetes
- Autoimmune conditions
- Heart disease
- Parkinson's disease
- High blood pressure
- Multiple sclerosis
- Thyroid imbalance
- Herniated discs
- Alzheimer's disease
- And more

Many people begin the therapy in order to treat one condition, such as arthritis, and they find that other conditions they have clear up as well. That's because the Gerson Method has proven effective for a wide variety of conditions – and that would be because so many of our health conditions directly relate to what we eat and what we are exposed to. When we remove those toxins and poisons from our bodies, they begin to function properly and without illness again.

Preventative Measures

In the rest of this book, we are going to take the time and focus on how to implement the Gerson Method in your own life to completely heal your arthritis. That's the purpose of the therapy – not to mask symptoms like so much of medicine does, but to help the body back to health.

The therapy is designed for people who are sick, and it will help them get well. If you are looking for a way to stay healthy, then you cannot use the method itself as a preventative measure.

However, you can follow the principles of the Gerson Method for good nutrition, and that will certainly help you stay healthy. These principles include the following:

- Only choose fresh, organic foods and that means nothing canned, preserved, GMO, or frozen.
- Cook vegetables by stewing them in their own juices so that they will retain their nutrients.
- The best vegetables for you are Brussels sprouts, artichokes, beets, carrots, peas, tomatoes, chard, spinach, red cabbage, cauliflower, and string beans.
- Salads are very good for you, especially when you combine mixed greens, tomatoes, carrots, celery, and cauliflower.
- Use plenty of fresh garden herbs for taste.
- Fruit, as long as it is fresh, is fantastic, so choose bananas, apples, applesauce, berries, oranges, grapefruit, grapes, and more. It's ok to choose some frozen fruits.
- Bake or boil potatoes. Do not fry them.
- Choose bread that is made with whole rye or whole wheat flour. Avoid anything refined.
- Eat plenty of oatmeal.
- For protein, choose fish, eggs, and nuts.
- Only drink a minimum amount of alcohol.
- Make sure you avoid these things: salt, nicotine, smoked fish, pepper, ginger, coffee, sodas, and caffeinated tea.
- Choose to drink herbal teas.

As you will learn later in this book, there are certain parts of the Gerson Method designed for healing arthritis. These include juicing and coffee enemas. These do not need to be included in any healthy diet. So, if you follow these rules for your healthy, preventative maintenance, then you should be able to maintain a much better life.

Now that we have discussed the Gerson Method and its history, along with how it could be used to heal other diseases and the guidelines it offers for a healthy life, we can move on to actually implementing the therapy so that your body can heal itself of arthritis no matter the type of the condition you actually have.

CHAPTER 4: RESTORING HEALTH

The journey to health has nothing to do with medication or trying to cover symptoms of your illness. Instead, it has to do with actually giving your body the tools it needs to heal itself. In fact, it is fully capable of healing without the need for any outside help.

Over the years, though, it has been deprived of the things it needs: nutrients, and it has been assaulted with toxins. According to the Gerson Method, nutritional deficiencies and toxicity are the two things that are keeping your body from healing itself.

Remember that, every single day, your body fights to be well. It wants to heal itself. That's because this is exactly what it is made to do. However, when it doesn't have the nutrients required to fight against illness, it cannot fight that fight. Additionally, when it is dealing with toxins constantly fighting against it, then the body constantly gets attacked by things that are making it sick.

So, the first steps of the Gerson Method will focus on getting your body moving in the right direction.

Hyperalimentation

When you are dealing with serious illness, then your body is essentially breaking down. You probably have noticed that you have lost your appetite, you are not eliminating properly, and you just feel bad. Because of this, you have to begin building your body back up. The best way to do this is through juicing and hyperalimentation. According to the

Medical Dictionary, this is:

> *"The ingestion or administration of greater than optimal amounts of nutrients." (Hyperalimentation, n.d.)*

Essentially, because your body has been deficient for so long, you have to go overboard for a while in order to get the nutrients back into your system.

Dr. Gerson found that the best way to do this is through juicing. So, the first thing you will need to do is follow the hyperalimentation diet. These are the parameters:

- You will need to eat three fully vegetarian meals a day. Ensure these meals include fresh, organic vegetables and prepare them only in their own juices.
- You will need to drink an eight-ounce glass of juice every hour. If you cannot drink all eight ounces, then you can cut the number down to four to six ounces and then slowly build up.
- Once you reach the point that you are able to consume all three vegetarian meals as well as 10-13 eight ounce glasses of juices every hour, then you will be able to move on to the next portion of the process.

The juicing process will depend on your condition, and different juices will be used in the Gerson Method depending on the illness.

- Carrots are often used in the juices because these vegetables are full of numerous healthy nutrients, including vitamin A, Potassium, protein, and fiber.
- Apples are an excellent source of potassium and other nutrients.
- Other juices have oxidizing enzymes, and these ingredients will help to make sure the blood stream is getting enough oxygen so that it can fend off illness.
- Oatmeal can be added to the juices to help ease digestion.

The great thing about the juices used in this process is that they can be adjusted depending on the person and their condition. For example, diabetics can be given juices that have lower sugar levels.

The main purpose of this portion of the method is to remove as much of the toxins from the body as possible while adding in required nutrients. Detoxification is a must because the toxins in your body are keeping you from getting well.

The Sodium Problem

Dr. Gerson understood that people have taste buds, and he knew that the beginning of this diet can be very difficult because of the lack of sodium. What you may not know is that you consume a high amount of sodium every single day without even realizing it. In the modern diet, sodium is in everything. It is used as a preservative and as a flavor. However, because of this, your taste buds become almost immune to every other flavor.

So, when you begin the Gerson Method, you may find that the food tastes boring, straw like or even cardboard like. It can be very difficult until your taste buds are able to adjust away from the salt. However, Dr. Gerson did provide a solution: you can use pressed, fresh garlic as much as you would like, which will come in handy when you eat your three daily meals. For the first few days, add as much garlic as you would like.

However, as your body adjusts and your taste buds are able to adjust through the deadening effect of sodium, you will find that you can actually enjoy the many flavors and characteristics of the foods you're now eating.

Here's a little secret: tastes are very strong in fresh, organic vegetables and fruits. You just cannot enjoy those flavors in the beginning. However, it should only take a couple of days for you to get those taste back.

The Importance of Rest

Do you know why you sleep? Of course, the most obvious reason for this would be that you sleep so that you can get over being sleepy. However, the whole reason why your body gets sleepy is that it needs time to heal and recover. That's the real purpose of sleep.

So, that's another problem that people have when they walk around sick. Not only are the toxins building up and the nutrients lacking, but also they are not getting the healing sleep their body needs. It's just a bad recipe.

This means the last part of the hyperalimentation process will be getting the rest and sleep that your body needs.

Here are a few guidelines that you will need to follow:

- Begin by going to bed around 10 pm. The later you stay up, the more you are depriving your body of the sleep and healing it needs.
- Make sure to take at least a one-hour nap every day after lunch.
- Get as much sleep as your body needs. Don't feel like you have to limit anything. If you are tired, you need rest.

During this process, there is a very good chance you will wake up through the night very thirsty. That's because your body is getting rid of toxins and that can create this excessive thirst.

You don't need to drink water at this time. Water will dilute the acids in your stomach, and that means your stomach will not be able to break down foods and extract the nutrients from them. Instead, when you find yourself thirsty, turn to peppermint or chamomile tea. These teas will promote rest, help to promote the acids in your stomach, and will even soothe the digestion process. Of course, they will ease the thirst you may be experiencing.

Detoxification

Another important part of preparing your body for healing will be detoxification. That's because right now, there is such a buildup of toxins within you that you simply cannot get well. Every day, you are exposed to:

- Additives
- Pesticides
- Cleaning Chemicals
- Other Toxins

As a result, your liver is no longer functioning properly. That's because the whole job of the liver is to remove toxins and cleanse the blood stream. However, when it is being flooded to such an extent, it simply cannot continue to work.

If you do not use the Gerson Method in the proper way described, then you could actually damage your liver. That's because there will be a rapid release of toxins as your body cleanses itself. If these toxins are not removed, the result can be poison to the liver that could do permanent damage.

That's why, in addition to the use of the proper diet, you must use coffee enemas as we will discuss later in this book. These enemas will remove the toxins from your body very quickly and ensure you do not have to worry about your liver. Removing these toxins will be an important first step in putting your body on the right path to healing, so make sure you detoxify your body as a part of the process.

As mentioned, we will go over the coffee enema process later in this book.

Exercise

Of course, as we mentioned, rest will be a very important part of healing, but exercise can be just as important. Even though you are going through the healing process and you may not always feel like it, exercise on some level is a must. This is especially true if you have conditions like obesity, high blood pressure, or diabetes.

The exercise should only be mild, however, and if you are unable to do anything right now, that is ok. You should never overextend yourself. It could cause more harm than good. Instead, you can bypass the exercise in order to allow your body to heal. Within just a few weeks, you should find that you will be able to engage in mild exercise very quickly.

Adding in Nutrients

In the first several days of this treatment, you will only need to follow everything that has been described above. That's because your body will not be able to handle the extra nutrients it actually needs. Adding them in too soon can cause digestive upset and make you feel very bad.

So, until your body has had time to adjust to the juices and the vegetarian meals, do not add in the supplements. However, once you have adjusted, there are several supplements that you will need. These include the following:

Potassium

When you are sick, you don't have enough potassium in your system. This mineral plays an important role of keeping too much salt from saturating into your cells. That can result in illness. So, one of the first supplements you should add in to your regular regime will be potassium.

Niacin

A supplement of this type will help to strengthen the liver by restoring glycogen levels. However, during the process of introducing niacin to your system, you may find that the capillaries, especially on your chest, may become red and even itchy. This is such a well-known side effect that it is called the "niacin flush". It is not dangerous and it will go away fairly quickly. When you add niacin to your supplements, do expect this side effect with the understanding that it will not last long.

Vitamin B12

The best way to get the vitamin B12 your body needs is to get a liver shot. This is an injection placed in the gluteus medius muscle and it is designed specifically to boost the liver health.

Keep in mind that as the liver contains all of the toxins your body is exposed to, it will become toxic itself. It is dangerous to your body and until you get your health sorted out, it needs to be the main focus of your healing. This shot will help to do this while giving your white and red blood cells the boost they need to provide healthy nutrients to the liver itself.

Lugol's Solution

This is a specialty solution that is designed to boost the health of your thyroid. This gland is very important in your body. It maintains your metabolism and controls your body heat. As a result, it has a massive impact on your immune system. A big part of your healing process will be ensuring that your body has a strong immune system and is strong enough to win the battle against illness.

This solution helps by improving the function of the thyroid gland and it is very easy to purchase in a health food store, a vitamin store, or online.

Dealing with Pain

Obviously, one of the biggest problems that comes along with arthritis will be pain, and that is why Dr. Gerson created something called the Triad specifically to help manage that pain while the body is healing. Once you begin this method and your body begins to recover, then this Triad may no longer be needed, but in the beginning, follow this formula:

- One Niacin tablet (50 mg)
- One Vitamin C tablet (500 mg)
- One regular Aspirin (325 mg)

You can take this combination every four hours throughout the day to manage your pain. As you continue through this Gerson Method, though, you should soon find that you no longer need it.

Everything we have discussed in this chapter will allow you to make the first steps toward healing through the Gerson Method. However, this is truly just the beginning. You will also have to make changes throughout your life, and that includes making sure everything in your household is Gerson compliant. That's what we will discuss in the next chapter.

CHAPTER 5: MAKING YOUR HOME GERSON FRIENDLY

There are many changes you will need to make in your household so that you can become healthy and follow the Gerson Method. Depending on how severe your condition may be, it can take up to two years or maybe even more to completely become well. Remember that you didn't get sick in just a few months. It took years and years, so keep in mind that it can take some time to get past that sickness.

So, even if you go to a Gerson treatment center, you will need to make changes within your household so that you can continue following the method when you go home.

The first thing you need to do is get rid of all of the toxic chemicals in your home. This includes pesticides, cleansing solutions, soaps with chemicals, and any tools that make things toxic, as well. Don't worry. You are going to replace all of these things with healthier and safer options. In the rest of this chapter, we are going to go over how you can create a healthy, Gerson-approved household.

Obviously, it will not matter if you remove toxins from your body if you turn around and reintroduce those same toxins in your own home. So, it is very important that you follow these steps.

The Kitchen

Obviously, the kitchen will be a very, very important space for your healing. That's because in the kitchen, you will be creating the juices and preparing fresh fruits needed so that you can become healthy. So, once you remove all of the toxins from your home (and that includes kitchen cleansers and other chemicals), then you can start equipping your kitchen with the things you will need so that you can follow this process properly.

Here is a list of equipment that you will need to make sure you have.

- Refrigeration – Since you will be keeping fresh, organic vegetables and fruits for all of your meals as well as your juices, you will need plenty of refrigeration space to store everything. Almost every type of fruit and vegetable will need to be kept in a refrigerator. It is recommended that you have a large refrigerator along with a couple of more medium sized ones.
- The Juicing – You will need two different things for juicing. The first of these is a good juicing machine. It will need to last for at least two years, so make sure it is a very durable model. Additionally, you will need a hand press so that you can press the pulp and get the remaining juice from it.
- The Oven – It can be very hard to ensure you have the right oven for cooking your vegetables. An electric model will not deplete oxygen in the home, but can be very hard to control as far as the heat intensity goes. A gas oven will be controllable, but will deplete oxygen, which is something you very much need to heal. The best option is to purchase a gas oven and then also install an ozone machine to produce more oxygen for the home. However, be very careful since the pure oxygen can be flammable.
- The Microwave – It is time to throw this out. We are a generation that expects convenience, and the microwave seems to offer just that, but this appliance is very bad for you in more than one way. To begin with, there are plenty of different research studies that indicate microwaves actually change the food on a molecular level and will completely remove anything good in those foods. Additionally, microwaves heat food unevenly and will actually create hot spots that can burn you. It is simply best to avoid the microwave at all costs.
- Pots – Aluminum is very bad for you. It has been linked to Alzheimer's disease and is certainly toxic for your body. When you use aluminum pots and pans, then this metal will be

transferred to your food every time you cook. So, you need to throw everything aluminum out and choose cooking materials like stainless steel, cast iron, and glass.

- Utensils – The same holds true of silverware. Do not use aluminum. Instead, choose stainless steel for your silverware and cooking utensils should be stainless steel or wood.
- Pressure Cookers – You should stop using this, too. While it may seem like a convenience, it can actually remove all nutrients from your food, as well. As you need to cook very slowly to ensure your meals are nutritious, a pressure cooker is a bad option.
- Water Filter – Although you will not be drinking water, you will need it for the enemas as well as for natural teas and cooking. The water you use needs to be free of all chemicals, including chlorine. The best way to ensure this is to buy a distiller, but you can also purchase distilled water if you would prefer.

Once you have your kitchen properly equipped, then you can move on to the next steps for your house.

Cleaning Supplies

Obviously, you need to keep your household clean since it will ensure you are free of germs and bacteria. However, cleaning supplies are filled with toxins and chemicals. You cannot buy those things from the store because they will only continue to make you sick. So, you have to start using cleaning supplies that have been approved for the Gerson Method to keep you safe from toxins and chemicals.

Here is a list of different things that are either approved or disapproved for use in your household.

Chlorine

Chlorine is used in almost any cleanser you can find for the kitchen and even for the rest of the home. It is also used freely in tap water and in swimming pools. The problem is, it is extremely toxic to the thyroid gland and can make you very, very sick. You must avoid it at all costs.

If you choose to purchase a commercial cleanser, then absolutely read through all of the ingredients and make sure there is no chlorine included.

Mix equal parts malt vinegar and water to create a cleaner you can use on kitchen and bathroom surfaces. Use white vinegar on other surfaces like wood.

Solvents

We think that we need solvents to keep things clean, but they are filled with harsh chemicals. You should avoid them at all costs, but if you find yourself in a situation where you must use a solvent, do so outdoors where it will dissipate and you will not be breathing it in.

Dishwashing Soap

This soap can include dangerous chemicals, but there is an easy way to ensure it is completely gone by the time you use a dish. In your dishwasher, it is normally set up to go through two wash cycles and one rinse. The thing is, since you will only be eating fresh vegetables, then you don't need that two wash cycle system. Instead, set the dishwasher to run through one wash cycle and two rinses. This will ensure all of the soap has been removed by the time you use the dishes.

Laundry Soap

For the most part, you should have no problem using laundry detergent as long as you make sure all soap is thoroughly rinsed from clothing before wear. It is a good idea to consider running your washing machine through two rinse cycles, as well. As long as you do this, you can even use bleach.

Fabric Softener

You will need to stop using fabric softener because it does leave a harmful chemical residue on your clothing. After all, the chemicals are so strong that many people are sensitive to it in the first place. You simply do not need to expose yourself to these chemicals. If you are very concerned with making your clothes soft, then consider adding distilled white vinegar to your washing machine. This will soften your clothes without the chemicals.

Aerosols

Obviously, these are no-nos. They put chemicals in the air and make it impossible for you to avoid breathing them in. It doesn't matter the product, you should always avoid aerosols, including bug sprays, cleansers, hair sprays, or anything else.

Window Cleaner

Any window cleaner can be very dangerous for you, and even if it is non-aerosol, you will still be breathing it in when it is sprayed in the air. The better way to clean your windows is to use white vinegar applied to a crumpled piece of newspaper.

While it may take some adjustments to get used to the new way of cleaning your home, it will certainly be worth it once you are healthy. You simply will no longer want those toxins in your home anymore.

The Bathroom

In the bathroom, you will have to look at things very carefully. That includes what you use to clean with and what you use to cleanse your body. As far as bathroom cleaners themselves, avoid anything that contains chlorine. Again, it is better to use white vinegar to clean surfaces.

As far as your body is concerned, the first thing you must remember is that your skin can soak in toxins. It is a permeable surface to some degree and that means you should choose carefully whenever you are going to put on your skin. You should choose only organic and chemical-free cleansers for the following:

- Cosmetics
- Aftershave
- Soap

- Shampoo
- Toothpaste
- Cream and Lotion
- Balms
- Deodorant
- Fragrances

Make sure you completely avoid any spray deodorants, hairsprays and other products. They will get in the air and you will breathe them in. As a result, you will be getting toxins into your body.

Thanks to a movement toward the organic, you can find these products available from many different sources, including local stores and online artisans.

When it comes to taking care of your teeth, dental hygiene is a must. You will have bacteria building up in your teeth and gums, and that bacteria could get into your bloodstream, which will turn toxic. However, you should not brush with any toothpaste that has fluoride in it. Again, look for an organic option, which will be available from many stores, shops, and artisans. Do not use baking soda to clean your teeth. It has sodium in it.

Make sure you rinse after brushing with distilled water, as tap water will have chlorine and other chemicals in it.

The Paint

During the healing process while you are on the Gerson Method of therapy, you should never paint in your home. It releases all sorts of chemicals into the air, and even if you leave windows open, the chemicals will get on your skin and into your lungs. If walls become dirty, wash them with plain soap and water.

Your Outdoor Areas

In your own property, do not use pesticides or any other type of spray. You will not be able to control what your neighbors may do, however, so if they use spray pesticides, then you will have to take extra steps to protect yourself. This would include keeping windows and doors shut and using an air cleaner or purifier. You need to limit your exposure to these chemicals as much as possible.

The Dentist

Before we finish up this chapter, here is an extra side note. If you have silver fillings in your teeth, then those fillings include small amounts of mercury. Even a very small amount of mercury, however, can be toxic. It has been connected with dementia and it will build up in your system, poisoning you. So, you should not:

- Have silver fillings placed
- Have silver fillings removed
- Have silver fillings cleaned or polished

It is important that you avoid these things during your treatment period. That's because even removing or cleaning a filling can release mercury into your mouth and therefore into your body.

Once you follow through with all of these things, your home will be prepared to ensure your Gerson Method therapy works. You do need to remove any toxins that your body can be exposed to, so go through your house and get rid of anything chemical in nature. Then, follow these rules for stocking, cleaning, and caring for your home.

If you go through every other part of the Gerson Method, but if you keep the chemicals in your home, then you will be defeating the whole purpose of the therapy. You cannot rid toxins from your body if you are surrounded by them as well. You won't be allowing the method to work and you will stay sick.

We have already discussed foods to an extent earlier in this book. However, in the next chapter, we will go into more detail on what foods you should include in your diet and what you should avoid.

CHAPTER 6: CHOOSING THE RIGHT FOODS

Food is one of the most important parts of the Gerson Method, and that is for very good reason. The things you put into your body will have a massive impact on what goes on with your health. If you consume toxins and poisons, then you are going to get sick.

When you consume things that your body actually needs, then you will be healthy. That's because your body is perfectly capable of healing itself. However, if it is lacking things or it is being filled with toxins, then it will not be able to do this.

The most important thing to remember about your food choices is this:

> *"Healthy eating is not about strict dietary limitations, staying unrealistically thin, or depriving yourself. Rather, it's about feeling great, having more energy, and stabilizing your mood." (Healthy Eating, n.d.)*

If you follow the dietary rules of the Gerson concept to stay healthy, then you will find that you are able to maintain a healthy weight and you will feel better. Even on the actual method for curing arthritis, you will not be so restricted that you waste away. That's not the purpose. Instead, the purpose is to provide you with the nutrients your body needs while ensuring you are not introducing toxins to your system.

Before we get into the actual foods that you cannot consume on the Gerson Method, let's look at a few rules. They really are actually quite simple.

- Sugar substitutes are toxic. They will make you sick, and that especially goes for aspartame, which is used in a variety of different "diet" products. Avoid Equal, NutraSweet, or any other sugar substitute of this nature.
- Salt is toxic for your body, yet it is constantly used in processed foods. You must avoid processed items for this very reason. If you don't want to ingest the toxins, then you have to avoid sodium.
- You must avoid industrial agricultural foods, like fruits and vegetables. These industrial offerings are sprayed with pesticides, chemicals to ensure they grow, and chemicals so that they will look good. Instead, you must choose all organic and fresh produce.
- All processed foods are bad, and that means you must avoid frozen, canned, packaged, jarred, microwaved, smoked, pickled, salted, or anything else. All of these processes include using additives that are toxic for your system.
- When you choose fruits and vegetables, do not take someone's word that they are organic. Only choose those items that have been certified organic. These will be the foods that have the nutrients your body needs without all of the toxins.

When you keep these rules in mind, then you will be able to make smart choices for your health, and these are the principles of the Gerson Method. It really does matter that you follow these rules very carefully. Breaking them even once or twice will reverse your progress and introduce poisons into your body.

Bad Foods

Now that we have gone over the basic rules, the next thing we need to discuss will be what foods you absolutely must avoid. This list is absolute. If you eat anything on this list, then you will be doing damage to your body, so if you intend to follow the Gerson Method and heal yourself of arthritis, then do not eat these foods:

- Alcoholic Beverages – You need to stop drinking alcohol completely.
- Avocadoes
- All Types of Berries – You can only have currants. The rest are no-nos.
- Baking Soda – This is often used in baking as well as in toothpastes. Eliminate it completely. Look for bicarbonate of soda on ingredients labels.
- Commercial Beverages – This refers to soda whether it is in a bottle or can.
- Sweet Things – Including cakes, chocolates, candies, and other confectionaries. They have no nutritional value and are filled with sugar and fat.
- Cheese – It contains dairy and as we discussed, dairy is very bad for you.
- Coffee – This is referring to drinking coffee specifically. We will discuss the importance of coffee enemas later.
- Cream – Again, this is a product that is made from dairy.
- Cucumbers – They do not digest very well and they are simply not the ideal option for your system.
- Dried Fruit – These processed versions of fruit are often glazed with oil or even contain sulfur.
- Water from the Tap – As mentioned, this contains chemicals including chlorine. You cannot have it in any form. So, you will need a distiller as discussed previously or you will need to buy distilled water specifically.
- Fats and Oils – The only oil you can have is flaxseed oil, and only in the amount that is prescribed to you by a Gerson specialist.
- Flour and Flour Products --- This includes breads, pastas, and cakes as well as anything that contains flour.
- Herbs – There are permitted herbs, but anything that is not on the good list will not be allowed.
- Ice Cream – Not only does it contain cream, but it also contains artificial sweeteners and additives.
- Sherbet – While it doesn't contain dairy, it does have additives

that are toxic.
- Beans (Legumes) – They will be added in to some degree later, but for the most part of the Gerson Method, you cannot have them.
- Milk – And that includes milk in all forms, whether it is fat free or not.
- Mushrooms – They are fungi and offer no nutritional value.
- Pickles – These are cucumbers that have been processed.
- Pineapples – They contain high amounts of aromatic oils that are not healthy for you.
- Nuts – While most people think they are healthy, nuts are too high in fat and they don't have the proteins your body actually needs.
- Soy – This includes all products made from soy, including milk, flour, tofu or anything else.
- Spices – This does not include garlic.
- Sprouts
- Sugar – And this means in any form, including refined white sugar and sugar substitutes.
- Tea – This doesn't include organic tea, but instead black or green, which contain caffeine and other additives. Some of them even include natural fluoride, which is a toxin.
- Wheatgrass Juice
- Butter – This is another product that contains dairy and is banned from your foods.
- Cottage Cheese – And that includes all forms, including fat free and salt free versions.
- Eggs
- Fish
- Other Types of Meats
- Yogurt – This would include any dairy product that is fermented.

There are probably a couple of things on that list which may surprise you a great deal because they are so highly touted for their nutritional benefits.

The two that may have surprised you the most are soy products and sprouts. Let's talk about them for a moment so that you can understand why consuming them is such a bad idea.

The Problems with Soy

You have probably heard over and over again that soy is so healthy for you that it is just the absolute best option for vegetarians so that they can get enough protein in their diet. The problem is, it is not healthy for you and can actually make you very sick.

- There is an oil in soy that is well-known for creating more than two dozen different allergic reactions, which can easily occur in many individuals.
- There is phytic acid in soy. This acid will keep your body from absorbing minerals that it needs to be healthy.
- There are enzyme inhibitors in soy. Enzymes are needed to keep your blood healthy and they are specifically included in the juices you will be drinking.

So, despite what you may have heard, soy is not good for you. It can make you sick and it can completely foil your attempts to be healthy.

The Problems with Sprouts

Since the health food craze began, plenty of people have flocked to natural food stores to buy sprouts and they eat them regularly on salads. You probably have been told over and over again that sprouts are a good option for you. However, they are completely banned from the Gerson Method. Surprised? Here's why you cannot have them. Studies from professionals of the Gerson Method show that sprouts are directly connected with actually developing illnesses including cancer.

The Problem with Wheatgrass Juice

Just as the health food movements have promoted sprouts, so too have they turned to wheatgrass juice as a healthy source of nutrients. While wheatgrass juice does have a lot of beneficial nutrients in it, it has problems as well. It is very hard to digest and will actually cause more harm than good. Additionally, the juices you will use on the Gerson Method will actually contain just as many nutrients while being very digestible.

It is very important that you follow these rules as far as foods you cannot have. Absolutely do not break the rules because they do have toxins in them in one way or another and they may not be easy to digest. The purpose of the Gerson Method is to give your body the tools it needs to heal itself, and that means getting the right nutrients while cutting out the toxins. Do this by avoiding the banned foods and eating the right things, which we will discuss next.

Citrus

Since you are seeking treatment for arthritis so that you can become well, you must avoid all citrus as it can have adverse effects. So, you will need to cut out limes, lemons, oranges, grapefruit, tangerines, etc.

Good Foods

After reading this list of things you cannot eat, you may have been completely shocked to the point that you are wondering what you can eat. Don't worry. There are plenty of healthy things you will be able to have in your diet. We have already discussed them somewhat earlier in this book.

This is actually a scary thought when you get right down to it. Consider this. If you read that list and thought you would have nothing to eat, then there's very good reason for this. You have been brought up in the modern world of processed foods. You have accepted all of the toxins and poisons. You have come to terms with the lack of nutrients. As a result, your body has suffered, but you have not seen this. It's not your fault, either. It simply has to do with the fact that you live in a world of convenience.

That's ok though because you are soon going to learn that there are foods available for you. Not only do they taste better, but they are good for you.

Your whole diet on the Gerson Method will be plant based, and that is a very good thing. Your body is made for plants, not meats. These foods contain healthy nutrients including enzymes, minerals, and vitamins. The meats you are eating right now don't contain those things, and whatever good they may have in them will actually be cancelled out by the poisons in them, as well.

Processed foods don't contain anything good for you. That's because the nutrients have been sucked out of them, and the processing added in a variety of toxins.

When you begin your journey into the Gerson Method, you will find that there is so much to discover with plant-based foods. Think about it when you visit the produce aisle. These foods are full of color and are full of flavor, as well. Your taste buds are about to embark on a wonderful journey and you are about to enjoy foods that you have never tasted before.

The main rule you need to remember when picking out foods is that they should be certified organic and you need to look for that specifically. Do not settle for signs that say the foods are organic. Make sure they actually are. That's because fruits and vegetables that are certified organic will not:

- Be exposed to pesticides
- Be grown from soil filled with chemicals
- Be genetically modified
- Be exposed to chemicals in fertilizers

Organic foods are fresh and natural, meaning they contain only nutrients and nothing bad for you.

Right now, you have all but killed your taste buds with salt and pepper as well as other seasonings. You don't know what it means to truly savor the foods that you eat. Instead, all you taste is that salt and all you expect is that salt. Since you will be removing sodium from your diet, you will be able to enjoy the true flavor of natural foods. At first, you may find foods bland, but soon, they will come out with all of their flavors and you will enjoy every single bite.

Here is a list of the preferred foods to include in your diet on the Gerson Method:

- Asparagus
- Green Apples
- Apricots
- Artichoke

- Arugula
- Beets
- Broccoli Tops
- Brown Sugar
- Horseradish (grated)
- Red Cabbage
- Carrots
- Cauliflower
- Celery
- Chard
- Cherries
- Chicory
- Chives
- Cilantro
- Corn (limited)
- Currants
- Eggplant
- Escarole
- Flax Oil
- Raisins
- Fresh Fruit
- Garlic
- Grapes
- Green Beans
- Honey
- Kale
- Leeks
- Lettuce
- Mangoes
- Melons
- Oatmeal
- Onions
- Parsley
- Peaches
- Pears
- Green and Red Bell Pepper

- Plums
- Potatoes
- Radishes
- Rhubarb
- Brown Rice (limited)
- Romaine Lettuce
- Rye Bread
- Allspice
- Anise
- Bay Leaves
- Coriander
- Dill
- Fennel
- Mace
- Marjoram
- Rosemary
- Sage
- Saffron
- Tarragon
- Thyme
- Sorrell
- Spinach
- Squash
- Sweet Potatoes
- Swiss Chard
- Tomatoes
- Red Wine Vinegar
- Cider Vinegar
- Watercress
- Yams
- Zucchini

In addition to those preferred foods, there are ones listed as limited. You can have them if they are allowed by your Gerson Therapy expert. They include:

- Quinoa – Only allowed once a week as a substitute for rice.
- Organic Popcorn – This should only be considered as a treat.
- Bananas – You can have one once a week.
- Maple Syrup and Molasses – Only a small amount once a day.

It's important that you understand what you can and cannot eat, so only have foods that are on this list.

Food Preparation

In addition to choosing the right foods, you will need to make sure they are prepared properly. The way you prepare your foods will have an impact on how nutritious they are for your body. If you cook them in the wrong way, then you will cook out all of the nutrients and you could actually add toxins to those foods.

Once you have properly equipped your home and your kitchen and have removed all of the banned foods, you will have everything you need to properly prepare your meals.

Here are some basic rules to follow as well as storing foods:

- Leafy greens do not keep well, so you will need to shop for them very often. Only buy small amounts that you can eat in a few days.
- Root vegetables as well as apples, pears, and oranges can keep for a much longer time so you are able to purchase them in larger amounts so that you don't have to shop for them as frequently.
- Make sure you have enough refrigerator space since you will be storing a large variety of vegetables and fruits inside.

When you prepare foods, there are a few rules you will need to follow as well. Keep in mind that you cannot cook foods at high temperatures. That's because these temperatures will actually destroy nutrients and take away the whole purpose of the food itself.

Additionally, you will not be able to use a microwave or pressure cooker because you will be removing nutrients and adding toxins. For the Gerson Method to work, you have to prepare your foods in a very specific way so that they will maintain their nutritional value.

The Preparation Method

When you prepare your foods for eating, then you will need to make sure you allow them to remain whole. That means do not peel them. You will be cooking them at a very low heat in their own juices so that they can maintain their nutrients.

Daily Menu

Breakfast

Breakfast on the Gerson Therapy always consists of a bowl of cooked oatmeal in distilled water. For variety, you can use a little honey, applesauce, dried or presoaked fruit.

Oatmeal is the exception (along with rye for the bread) for all grains that is permitted. The water-soluble fiber is very valuable, and helps to cushion the juices coming down the pike. It provides soft bulk to help move the contents of the intestines along. That does NOT mean that all grains are good and consumable; only that oatmeal's benefits outweigh its properties as a grain.

Lunch

Treating arthritis alternatively involves eating Gerson's Hippocrates Soup recipe that heals and strengthens the immune system and kidneys.

Ingredients:

- 1 medium celery knob or 3-4 stalks of celery
- 1 medium parsley root – if available
- Garlic as desired
- 2 small leeks (if not available, replace with 2 medium onions)
- 1 ½ pounds tomatoes or more
- 2 medium onions
- 1 pound of potatoes
- A little parsley

Directions:

1. Do not peel any of these special soup vegetables
2. Wash and scrub them well
3. Cut them coarsely
4. Simmer them slowly for 2 hours
5. Then put them through a food mill in small portions
6. Only fibers should be left
7. Vary the amount of water used for cooking according to taste and desired consistency.
8. Keep well covered in refrigerator no longer that 2 days
9. Warm up as much as needed each time

Additionally, eat a salad with the soup. Just mix different types of lettuces, onion and celery.

After the soup and the salad, you can make mashed potatoes if you're still hungry.

Dinner

Dinner is the same as lunch. But don't eat potatoes this time. Eat fruits.

The Juices

One of the most important steps in the Gerson Method is juicing. This will be the groundwork for the rest of the therapy. When you begin the Gerson Method, you will be drinking around 13 glasses of juice a day and this is the best way to cleanse your body of toxins and get the nutrients you need.

There are only four different juices that will be used and they are actually the same options used to treat any illness on the Gerson Method with one exception. They include:

- Apple/Carrot – You should wash approximately eight ounces of apples and carrots and then brush them to remove debris. Do not peel them. Place them in the juicer whole.

- Carrot Only – The carrots need to be washed and brushed but not peeled. Make sure you grind about 10-12 ounces and then press through the juicer.
- Apple Only – In other Gerson treatments, such as for cancer, citrus will be used. However, for arthritis patients, citrus should be avoided. Just wash and brush clean about eight ounces of apples, grind, and press.
- Green Juice – For this juice you will need: romaine lettuce, red leaf lettuce, endive, escarole, red cabbage, inner beet tops, green pepper, Swiss chard, watercress, and apple. Grind everything thoroughly before pressing. If you cannot get some of these items, leave them out and do not try to replace.

These are the juices you will use on a daily basis, so be sure to keep a stock of the organic, fresh fruits and vegetables you will need.

The very idea of juicing can be confusing for some people and may raise quite a few questions.

Why Not Just Regular Food?

There is a reason for every part of the Gerson Method. When you drink eight ounces of fresh juice every single hour of the day, then you will be consuming as much as 17 pounds of fruits and vegetables in a day.

Now, take a moment and imagine eating that many pounds of food. It would be impossible! And, it probably turns your stomach even thinking about it. Your body must have all of those nutrients so that it can begin functioning properly, but since you cannot consume that much food, you can get those things through juices.

That's not the only reason why juicing is so important. Many people who use this therapy do so because they are very, very sick. Whether you are sick from arthritis or something else, juicing will help you get better without making you feel bad. All of the toxins in your body will mess up your digestive system.

You probably don't have enough stomach acid. Your digestive tract is full of poisons. If you try to eat everything without juicing, you will not be able to digest the foods properly. It will be rough on your system. Juices, though, don't cause these problems.

Why Can't I Make Juice and Store It?

Some people wonder if they could save some money by simply making up a batch of juice and keeping it in the refrigerator. That seems like a good idea, but it actually is not. There is a vastly different response in the body when you drink juice that is even a couple of hours old versus if you drink juice that is fresh. There are lots of theories why this is the case:

Fresh juice can actually be absorbed into the body before it reaches the stomach. Essentially, enzymes can make their way into the body thanks to membranes in the mouth and esophagus. Juice that is older will not be able to do this.

Juice that is more than an hour old will lose its vital force. Plants and vegetables all have a vital force that transfers energy to you, as well. When you drink fresh juice, you are drinking the vital force and this will help your body heal. If you consume juice that is older, then you will lose that vital force.

When juice is made fresh, it has a high liquid content, and that liquid will allow the kidneys to flush properly so that toxins can leave the body. If juices sit for very long, then a lot of the liquid will evaporate.

So, this is why you need to make sure you are making fresh juices. Your body needs all of the nutrients and healing it can get, and fresh juice will allow this to happen.

This is especially the case with the green juice. Never store it and always drink it right away after making it. The carrot/apple juice can actually be stored for up to 72 hours, but this isn't recommended.

If you do need to store the juice, do so in small jars, eight ounces each if possible. You don't want any room in the jar where air can stay. Instead, it needs to be sealed tight and air free. Don't use a larger container for storage because you will have to open it too many different times.

Can I Add in My Own Vegetable and Fruit Choices?

No, you cannot. Each of the juices you will drink while on the Gerson Therapy have been selected for their nutritional value and their healing abilities. So, when you are on this therapy, follow the juice mixtures exactly, and that means no substitutions or additions.

Can I Drink Water Instead of Juices?

Water should not be added to your diet at all. Water will dilute the acids within your stomach and will actually slow down your healing process. Additionally, water can dilute the nutrients in the juices. As a result, you will not get the healing you need. When you drink the juices themselves, you are getting the liquids you need. So, don't worry. You will not become dehydrated.

In some instances, such as at night when you wake up with stomach upset, then you can drink organic teas, including peppermint or chamomile. However, all other water should be removed from your diet.

Why Can't I Use Red Apples?

When you begin the Gerson Therapy, you should only use Granny Smith apples. This is a specific rule. Red apples don't have the same nutrients.

If you cannot get Granny Smith apples and you need a substitute, it needs to be another tart green apple, like the Fuji. It is always best to use the Granny Smith, so do your best to get those. Do not ever use red apples in your juices.

Why Can't I Use Raw Spinach?

Many people think that spinach is very healthy for them, so they may consider adding it to their diet on the Gerson Method. However, you cannot do this. Spinach itself will actually inhibit your body from absorbing nutrients from other foods, so you do not need it in your diet.

What Happens If I Cannot Get Organic Ingredients?

For some people, it could be hard to get fresh, organic foods, and you may think it is ok to use other fruits and vegetables, but that is not the case. No matter what, when you purchase the produce, you cannot purchase anything unless it is organic. Any of that produce could be filled with pesticides and chemicals and it will introduce toxins into your body.

You cannot take that risk.

If for some reason you are not able to get a certain organic ingredient, the best option is to leave it out of your juices until you can get it again. Do not try to make substitutions or you could make a big mistake and derail your healing process.

Food is also important to your healing with the Gerson Method, so the more you understand how to follow the rules, you will be able to gain success. What you must remember is that changing any of this even the least little bit will ruin your progress. Anything non organic will have toxins in it. Anything on the banned list will only make you sicker.

When you finish the Gerson Therapy, there are certain ways you can loosen up your diet routine, which we will discuss later in this book, but for now, you must follow these rules so that the method can actually work to remove toxins from your body and add in the nutrients you need.

Once you begin the Gerson Method, and if you follow the rules, then your body will be given the tools it needs to heal itself. It's as simple as that.

CHAPTER 7: ENEMAS FOR THE GERSON METHOD

In addition to the food, the second major point of the Gerson Therapy will be coffee enemas. This is probably the most difficult part of the method for you to grasp, especially if you are just now learning about this therapy.

Obviously, there has been plenty of criticism of the coffee enema, but there is actually scientific backing for this process, and it is integral to the Gerson Method. Without the coffee enema, the method itself will not work.

What They Are

When you begin eating according to the Gerson Method, your body will begin flushing toxins out of it, but those toxins can settle into the lower digestive tract. So, eating the right food is only the first step. The second step is to completely flush those toxins from the rest of your body.

That's not the only part of the coffee enema. It also introduces nutrients into the body and helps to ensure hydration.

One important thing to remember is that coffee enemas have been around a very long time. They have been used for hundreds and hundreds of years in order to provide hydration. In fact, even in the modern day, enemas are regularly used in hospitals to irrigate the colon and remove toxins. So, it should be no surprise that coffee enemas can be helpful, and are a very important method used in the Gerson Method.

The Four Purposes of the Coffee Enema

Let's look at the four purposes of the coffee enema specifically.

Remove Toxins

As we mentioned, removing toxins from your body is a very important step in the Gerson Method. Without eliminating toxins, your body cannot heal itself because it is being poisoned. The coffee enemas work together with the change in diet to completely flush the system.

Cleansing the Colon

The large intestine and colon can have a variety of different toxins in them. For example, when things do not digest in the proper way, they may stay within the colon, turning into rot and fermented sugars. It is a poison. The coffee enema will help to flush away those things from the large intestine and will work with astringent properties.

Stimulating Bile Flow

Bile is an important part of the body and the digestive system. Many of the toxins you may be ingesting will actually block bile flow and that can make you very sick. Coffee enemas will actually increase the amount of bile flow your body is able to produce, and when bile is flowing properly, even more toxins will be flushed from the body.

Stimulating a Healthy Liver

As we have already discussed, when toxins build up in your body, they poison your liver. Even after removing the toxins, your liver is damaged and sick. It will need time to heal itself and coffee enemas can help it do so.

So, as you can see, it doesn't matter how surprised you may be to read about coffee enemas, you should know that they are very helpful and a very important part of getting well. If you don't follow this protocol, then the whole Gerson Method will not work.

Still Unsure?

Some are still unsure of whether or not coffee enemas can actually work. However, as mentioned, there are scientific backings that show how this treatment can be successful.

Here are a few of the studies that have been done that show how helpful coffee enemas can actually be.

- In the 1920s, a study was done in Germany in which rats were infused with caffeine. The results of this study found that caffeine reaches the liver through the hemorrhoid vein and this will allow the bile ducts to clear out and release bile so that everything will flow properly. Additionally, ingredients in the caffeine allow the blood vessels to dilate and the muscles to relax.
- A study that was conducted at the University of Minnesota found that coffee, when administered through the rectum, will actually stimulate the enzyme system, especially in the liver. This means that free radicals (which are very dangerous) are destroyed before they cause cellular damage.

So, yes, studies have shown that the Gerson Method and coffee enemas actually work. They aren't just an idea. They are actually proven ways to clear the body of toxins and poisons.

Here are just a few of the things you can expect to happen when you use coffee enemas regularly as prescribed by the Gerson Therapy. Patients will:

- Enjoy increased cell production, which means your body will be able to replace damaged, sick cells for a healthier system.
- Experience healthier tissues.
- Notice improved circulation in the blood stream.
- Enjoy a better, stronger immune system.
- Experience quicker cellular regeneration.

Those are the benefits of the coffee enemas for the purposes of the Gerson Method, but they actually have some positive side effects, too. For example, patients who use them regularly and as prescribed find that the enemas help to relieve pain and digestive upset while easing tension and even reducing the effects of depression.

A Word of Warning

You have probably noticed that quite a few celebrities have been using something called high colonics as a way to supposedly be healthy. While this has become the newest fad, it is certainly not something you should be doing. It is not safe and it is not something you need to include in your Gerson Therapy. High colonics are actually dangerous because they can cause the intestine to distend. Not only does the water in high colonics wash away anything bad, but it will also flush away enzymes, nutrients, and minerals that your body needs. You will lose the good bacteria your body needs to digest properly.

Coffee enemas are different. They allow the liver to release toxins and they do not flush away healthy things your body needs.

How to Use Them and How Often

Right now, you have a lot of toxins in your body, and for that reason, you will need to partake in coffee enemas at least five times a day. That may seem like quite a bit, but this is the only way to truly detoxify. Each enema will be held within the body for around 12-15 minutes and that way, all of your body's blood will pass through the liver several times. That way, it will have the most exposure to detoxification.

The first thing you need to do is get the right coffee and equipment. Here are a few rules you need to keep in mind:

- You need a source of distilled water or filtered water. It must not contain chlorine.
- The right coffee will be all organic. It should be a medium to light roast coffee at a medium drip grind.

In addition to those two things, you will need the right enema equipment, which is not as simple as going to the store and buying it. There are things you need to keep in mind when purchasing it.

The kinds of enema equipment you will see readily on hand at the store, like combination syringes and rubber bottles, will actually not suit your purposes very well. For one thing, they are very hard to clean. For another thing, they can wear out very quickly with regular use.

The best option will be a bucket enema. The buckets will include a measuring system and connections for your tubing and supplies. You can choose between stainless steel and plastic. Plastic is usually clear so that you can see the progress of the enema but it can be broken easily. Stainless steel isn't clear, but it will last longer.

Make sure you replace the rubber tubing from time to time so that your enema equipment will remain clean and sanitary.

Preparing Your Enema

You will find it much easier to go ahead and mix up everything for your enema for the whole day. That way, you won't have to go through this process every four hours. Here is what you need to do.

1. Measure out three full tablespoons of coffee and add it to a small pot.
2. Add 32 ounces of water.
3. Mix thoroughly and bring the mixture to a boil. Keep it at a rolling boil for three minutes and then simmer for another 15 minutes.
4. Strain the mixture through a cloth strainer or something very fine.
5. Add back water until you have one quart of mixture.
6. This mixture is for one enema, but you can mix it up for the whole day by multiplying all ingredients and using a bigger pot.
7. Make sure the enema mixture is at body temperature when used.
8. Clamp the tube shut and then pour the mixture into your enema bucket.
9. Unclamp the tube just a small amount in order to allow all air to be evacuated from the tube.
10. Eat a small bit of fruit before starting the enema. This will boost the digestive system and this is especially important first thing in the morning.

Now, you will be prepared to use your enema. Just make sure the solution is at least at body temperature before you use it.

Using the Enema

When it comes to using your enema, it will work the best if you are relaxed and comfortable. So, you need to create the right space so that you will be at complete ease during the whole process. You should probably use the enema in the bathroom, so you will need to create a comfortable spot on the floor. Do this with:

- A soft blanket
- An enema mat or shower curtain to manage any spills
- A comfortable cushion for your head
- A stool or hook for the bucket to be hanged about 18 inches above you

Once you have all of this in place, you will be ready to administer your enema. Make sure you use Vaseline to lubricate a couple of inches of the tubing tip. Then, insert the tip into the rectum before releasing the clamp.

Once you have released the clamp, then you will need to lay on your side with your legs pulled toward your chest. You can call it curling up or laying in the fetal position. No matter what, remember to continue breathing deeply and stay relaxed. You may even wish to play soothing music, choose this time to meditate, or read a relaxing book. You will need to retain the coffee solution for around 12-15 minutes. Then, it can be evacuated.

Patients who have serious illnesses like cancer will need to do coffee enemas more often, but for your treatment of arthritis, you only need to do the coffee enemas three times a day. That will give you an idea of how much of the solution you need to prepare every morning.

Keeping Everything Clean

You will need to make sure you keep all of your equipment clean so that it is safe for use. You don't have to sterilize the equipment because it is used in an unsterile place. However, you do need to clean it. After every use, wash out the bucket and all of the tubing with warm, soapy water. Make sure you flush all of the soap out.

A few times a week, place hydrogen peroxide in the bucket and leave it for several hours or overnight. You just need to make sure you rinse everything thoroughly after doing that.

Preparing for Complications

A coffee enema is completely healthy and safe. It will work wonders for you in conjunction with the Gerson Method diet. However, as with anything to do with your body, there is always a chance of complications. It is a good idea to prepare for any side effects that could arise so that you will not be scared if they do happen.

The most important thing to keep in mind is that these complications have nothing to do with the enema itself, but instead to do with conditions your body was already in. Don't make the mistake of thinking you should stop using the enema. Let's address some of the things that can happen.

- For many people who are on medications for their illness, their digestive system may become sluggish. As a result, they could have an impaction and they may not be able to take in all of the enema or hold it for the full time. That's ok if this occurs. Just take in as much of the enema as you can and hold it for as long as you can. Soon, the impaction should resolve itself.
- If you have gas retention, this could keep the enema from working. If this is the case, then you will need to follow this procedure: Allow a part of the coffee solution to flow in, then lower the bucket to your body level. This will allow the enema to flow back into the bucket and you may notice bubbling as the gas is released. When this happens, you can re-raise the bucket to complete the enema.
- Because you are using the Gerson Method for arthritis, you may find it uncomfortable or painful to lie on your side. If that is the case, then lie on your back and raise your knees to your chest as much as possible.
- If you have severe bowel inflammation, then the coffee enema can be too strong for your system. Try reducing the coffee levels and mix with chamomile tea as opposed to water. Additionally, you can add in a pure chamomile enema in the mornings to soothe your digestive system.

Many of these issues will clear up as you move forward with the Gerson Method. That's because your body is going through the healing process. It will take time for everything to straighten out. As the toxins flush from your system, you will find that you feel better and the enemas go smoothly, as well.

We will discuss another type of enema problem later in this book, called flare-ups, and you will learn how you can treat this problem so that it doesn't cause issues. In the next chapter, we will begin discussing medications because there are certain ways you can medicate yourself in a healthy and natural way so that the Gerson Method will work better as well.

CHAPTER 8: WHAT YOU NEED TO KNOW ABOUT MEDICATION

What do you think of when you hear the word, "medication"? You probably imagine a prescription given to you by the doctor or something you can pick up over the counter at your pharmacy. What you are imagining isn't truly a medication at all, though. Instead, it is a mask. It covers up your symptoms, but does not make you better.

You have to throw away your conventional concept of medication and understand what we describe in this chapter is true medication; things that will actually help your body heal and not just make you feel better. These medications will help you heal and that will make you feel better too.

Think about this. How many times have you taken something you got from a pharmacy – something that was supposed to make you feel better – only to discover that you have to deal with many different severe side effects. Sometimes, you even have to take other medications in order to deal with those side effects. It is a never ending cycle, and it is one that will not help you get well.

When you consider the things we call medicines here, they don't cause side effects. They are completely natural supplements that will help make you well, not make you sicker. So, for you to understand how these medicines can be used and how they will help you as you go through the Gerson Method, we should go through your options and explain each of them.

Potassium

Because you have been consuming a diet very high in sodium, your cells have become damaged, and that sodium keeps your body from getting the potassium it needs. Potassium is an absolute must for your health, and a lack of it can contribute to degenerative conditions like diabetes. The first of these medications is one that will work specifically to help you heal from arthritis. It is a compound.

You will need to dissolve 100 grams of potassium salts in distilled water. You will need to store this compound in a dark place. If you don't have a dark bottle, then you can wrap it in a paper bag.

Then, mix about four tablespoons of the compound into your juices for the day. Make sure you do this for all ten of your juices. As the compound works, you can reduce the mix to two tablespoons for each of the ten juices a day.

Depending on how ill you are, you may find that your potassium balances out in a few weeks, months, or years. You just need to make sure you keep using the compound until your body is no longer deficient.

Lugol's Solution

We have already discussed Lugol's Solution to an extent, but let's look at it one more time.

When you drink water from the tap, you are exposing yourself to chlorine and fluoride. These remove iodine from your thyroid gland, and iodine is much needed for proper function. Over time, your thyroid cannot do what it is supposed to, and, as a result, your metabolism drops, which means:

- You feel tired and sluggish
- You gain weight very easily
- You don't have energy to exercise
- You find yourself irritable

When your metabolism is low, your whole system is off-balance. That's not the only problem that will arise when your thyroid is not functioning properly, either. It is the thyroid that controls body temperature and tells your body when you have an infection. That's why you get a fever when you are sick. This means your immune system will not work properly.

Lugol's Solution is designed to restore function to the thyroid and to ensure you have a higher metabolism and immune system. Blood tests will need to be performed by a doctor in order to ensure your thyroid is functioning properly after you have been using Lugol's Solution for some time.

Niacin

You probably have heard of niacin plenty of times before. After all, it shows up in multivitamins and even in some of the foods you were regularly eating. However, the damage that came along with those packaged foods means the niacin you were getting just wasn't helpful. Now that you have begun the Gerson Method, you may need a niacin medication.

It accomplishes a number of different things, including:

- Aiding in digestion of proteins
- Improving blood circulation
- Ensuring oxygenated blood gets to all of the tissues in the body
- Reducing excess water that is retained in the abdomen
- Relieving many types of abdominal pain

Niacin can be extremely helpful in your healing process. So, if you need to add this to your treatment, then here is what you will need to do:

During meals, you will need to take one 50 mg pill five times a day. As we discussed earlier in this book, you may experience the niacin flush, but it will go away and it is not dangerous. So, do not stop your niacin regimen just because you experience the flush.

Liver Medications (Capsules and Injections)

Your liver will be severely damaged from all of the toxins and poisons you have ingested. The liver is designed to filter out toxins, but when it becomes overly taxed, it simply can no longer do the job. For that reason, a couple of the medications that you may need to take on the Gerson

Treatment will focus on healing the liver and restoring its functionality.

- Liver Pills – The first of these medications is a capsule. This capsule will contain dried and powdered liver from animals. It will need to be taken three times a day when you are drinking carrot juice specifically.
- Liver Injections – The second option is a liver injection, which also contains Vitamin B12 and will help patients who have become anemic with their illness. Not only has this medication shown to heal anemia, but also it has shown to help fend off degeneration of the bones and joints, especially in the spine. This medication is given as a 3 cc injection into the muscle. In the beginning, it will need to be administered every other day. As the liver begins to heal, the frequency can be reduced.

Your liver is so important to your well-being, and when it starts shutting down, toxins will build up in your body. You will have no defense from those toxins and they will only make you sicker. While you use the diet and the coffee enemas to flush the toxins from your body, you will also need to take care of your liver, and that means using medications such as these to heal this important organ.

Pancreatin

The pancreas performs an important job in digestion. It creates enzymes that will break down fats, sugars, and certain types of protein. Obviously, you don't ingest these things when you are on the Gerson Method. That doesn't mean, however, that you no longer need those enzymes. You have to take care of your pancreas, as well, and this is especially true if you have atherosclerosis (hardening of the arteries). That's because this enzyme helps to break down the plaque in your arteries so that your heart can function properly.

Pancreatin is a medication that will help ensure your pancreas is working properly, and it will help aid in digestion as well. To take this medication, you will need to have three 325 mg tablets four times a day. You can take them after each meal and then sometime in the mid-afternoon.

Acidol Pepsin

This is a medication that is used to specifically help induce an appetite. Many patients who are very sick don't have a strong appetite just because their bodies are so poisoned. In those cases, this medication can be used. However, there are certain times when it should not be administered.

- If the patient has acid reflux, then the medication should not be used.
- If the patient has stomach ulcers, they should not take this medication.
- If the patient has stomach lining irritation or inflammation, they should not use this medication.

In these cases, acidol pepsin can actually upset your stomach even more. However, in other cases, it can certainly improve appetite so that the patient can eat the meals and drink the juices as prescribed by the Gerson Method.

Flaxseed Oil

This oil is full of essential fatty acids that your body needs to be well. These include Linoleic acid and linolenic acid. These two help your body in several different ways. Flaxseed oil also contains high amounts of omega three fatty acids, which your body also needs. This medication is used for several purposes and will help by:

- Ensuring the cells and cell membranes are getting the oxygen they need to be healthy and repair themselves.
- Removing, dissolving, and ridding the body of toxins that are fat soluble.
- Ensuring Vitamin A gets to the body so that it can boost the immune system.
- Reducing cholesterol levels for a healthier body and healthier arteries.

This is a medication that should be used only as prescribed. You cannot take as much as you would like. Instead, you should start out with two tablespoons every day. Do this for a month and then reduce the dosage to one tablespoon per day.

CoQ10

This is a medication that has only been added to the Gerson Method very recently because it is a fairly new treatment that people have only recently learned about. Coenzyme Q10 replaces nutrients that your body desperately needs.

Here are some facts about CoQ10:

- When you are deficient in it, you may experience a variety of different illnesses, including chest pain, high blood pressure, and even heart failure.
- When used as a regular supplement, CoQ10 can actually reverse the symptoms of heart failure.
- CoQ10 can have a massive effect on high blood pressure to relieve stress on the heart and veins.
- This medication can even reduce and reverse age related macular degeneration. This is a type of vision loss.
- CoQ10 has shown to be effective in slowing the progression of Alzheimer's disease.
- Studies have shown that the medication can help slow the progress of ALS.
- The medication, when combined with other vitamins, has been beneficial to easing the symptoms of asthma.
- CoQ10 is an antioxidant, which means it will help to flush toxins from the body and build a stronger heart.
- When the body is deficient in CoQ10, this has been linked to breast cancer in women. In addition, higher levels of CoQ10 have even been shown to increase the survival rate of patients who have been diagnosed with end stage cancer.
- The medication has been shown to help reverse cataracts.

This is just the beginning, too. The medication has shown to be beneficial in reversing the effects of such diseases as:

- Chronic Fatigue Syndrome
- Side Effects of Chemotherapy
- Chest Pain (angina)
- Coronary Heart Disease
- Cystic Fibrosis
- Dry Mouth
- Fibromyalgia
- Gum Disease
- Hearing Loss
- Heart Disease
- High Cholesterol
- HIV and AIDS
- Kidney Failure
- Migraines
- Infertility
- Mitochondrial Disease
- Mitral Valve Prolapse
- Muscular Dystrophy
- Parkinson's Disease
- Pre-Eclampsia
- Psoriasis
- Prostate Cancer
- Tinnitus
- Diabetes
- Hepatitis C
- Huntington's Disease
- Cocaine Dependency

As you can see, CoQ10 has a lot of benefits, and it certainly could be used to help your health even if you aren't currently going through the Gerson Method. If you are going through the method, though, you will need to follow these dosing instructions:

- Take one 50 mg pill per day for five to seven days
- Increase to 100 mg per day for a week
- Continue increasing until you reach 600 mg per day.

It is important to follow this method because some people are particularly sensitive to CoQ10 and they may become sick from taking too much too quickly.

Anytime you take medications on the Gerson Method, it should be one of these, and it is best to do so with the supervision of a Gerson expert. That's because some people are sensitive to different types of medications, especially CoQ10, and they will need to be handled properly.

Medications will take on a fully different meaning now that you are using the Gerson Therapy. You do not need to take those toxic medicines that you could buy over the counter or with a prescription. If you take those things, you are introducing toxins into your body. The medications described here don't make you sick or just mask your illness. Instead, they actually help you heal when used properly along with the rest of the Gerson Method.

In the next chapter, we are going to discuss something very important: the reactions your body may have whenever it begins to heal.

CHAPTER 9: HEALING REACTIONS

You took a long path to get where you are physically. Over all of the years of your life, you have been exposed to toxins and poisons. You have been exposed to illness, injury, and damage. It's a path that has led you to where you are right now. Maybe you have arthritis in your knee and you have always been told it was due to an old sports injury. Maybe the arthritis in your hands has set in and you were told it's because your body is attacking itself. No matter the case, the actual reasons for your condition are deficiencies of nutrients and toxicity in your body.

What you must remember is that it didn't happen overnight. The road is long and winding. When you use the Gerson Method to heal your body, you will have to go through that process in reverse. Your body has to go through all of those steps in reverse to get back to true health. That means, then, you will experience something called healing reactions.

> *"Healing reactions are temporary symptoms that occur as a result of the retracing process. Most of the time, they go unnoticed, although some can be unpleasant, and rarely they are frightening or even dangerous. As a rule, however, the body will not retrace or begin a healing reaction unless it can see it through to completion." (Wilson, 2014)*

Healing reactions may be scary at times, but they are good things.

That's because they signify that your body is healing itself. They are also called flare-ups, as we mentioned earlier in this book. They can be scary if you don't expect them. That's because you will think you are getting worse. You aren't, though. Your body is healing.

Since they are inevitable with the Gerson Method, let's discuss them in more detail. First, let's go over a few facts:

- Flare-ups are almost always safe, although scary. Do not stop your therapy just because you have a flare-up.
- The first flare-up you may experience will be relatively short. That's because your body will not yet be in a position to fully heal itself. Instead, it will be weak and the fighting it does against toxins and deficiencies will result in a flare-up for a short time.
- If you only have arthritis and no other serious condition, then your flare-ups will be fairly mild compared to someone who has serious illness like cancer.
- There is no way to put a time frame on how long each flare-up will last. The first will be mild, but after that, it will all depend on your body and how many toxins must be flushed away.
- If you stop the treatment, you will end up becoming sick again. You cannot stop the Gerson therapy just because you have a healing reaction.

While you cannot stop the flare-ups and you should recognize them as a sign of healing, you will also find that they can be quite unpleasant. For that reason, you need to understand what you can do in order to ease the symptoms of healing reactions.

Blood Clots

First of all, when you begin the Gerson Method, it won't just heal your arthritis. Your body is not a selective healer. It will heal everything wrong within it, from allergies to scars. For that reason, as your body heals, the calcium buildups within your arteries, called atherosclerosis, will begin breaking up and dissolving in the bloodstream. During that time, there is a very slight chance of blood clots. However, for as long as the Gerson Method has been used, there has been no sign that these blood clots could cause any problem.

For that reason, blood thinners are never recommended while you are on this treatment. Instead, if blood clots were to form, they should pass through your bloodstream and out of your system with no trouble whatsoever.

Nausea

This is a very common symptom of healing reactions when you are on the Gerson Method for arthritis. There are several different things you can do to ease the nausea depending on the severity of the flare-up.

To begin with, you should always continue juices while you are dealing with the flare-up. However, if you find that you cannot stand to drink them, then you will need to consider enemas. This can be done especially with the green juice and any juice in fact (except for orange juice which you will not be drinking on the arthritis therapy anyway). There are a few rules, however:

- This is called an implant enema. You will retain the juice after the enema, which means do not expel it.
- Make sure the juice has reached body temperature. The best way to do this is to let it stand or float in warm water.
- Once the juice has been administered as an enema, you can lay in a comfortable bed and pull your legs up to your chest. You need to stay there until the juice has been absorbed into the body.

If you are unable to drink the juices and must use the enema method, then you will also need to do things to settle your stomach and ensure you are getting the liquids you need. This includes drinking oatmeal gruel and peppermint tea.

Oatmeal Gruel

To make oatmeal gruel, you will need organic oatmeal, a small saucepan, and a strainer. Begin by mixing one ounce of oats with five ounces of water and allow the mixture to come to a boil. Then, lower the temperature and allow the mixture to simmer for 10 minutes.

Run the mixture through a very fine strainer so that all you are left with is a thick liquid. Make sure to press the oats in the strainer to get as much liquid as possible. Drink the mixture while it is warm. This will help settle your stomach, will ensure you get the liquids you need, and will not dilute your stomach acids.

If you find that you are not able to stand any of your juices because your stomach is so upset, then top two ounces of oatmeal gruel with six ounces of the juice and drink this instead.

Peppermint Tea

Peppermint tea is especially helpful if you have an upset stomach because the peppermint itself will relieve nausea. However, even if you are not sick to your stomach, you can use this tea simply if you are thirsty. It's a useful thing to keep in a thermos and have available on your nightstand if you wake up thirsty or nauseated during the night.

For peppermint tea, you can use fresh peppermint or fresh spearmint. Add a large tablespoon of the leaves to boiling water and allow to steep for 15 minutes before straining.

So, if you are nauseated, then try these things. They will make a big difference, and remember that the healing reaction is only temporary.

Stomach Problems

Diarrhea is a common healing reaction during the Gerson Method. You should not be alarmed if you deal with bouts of it on a regular basis, but it is uncomfortable, so there are ways you can treat the condition so that you will be more comfortable.

- If you experience diarrhea, then stop juices for the time being and drink 5-6 glasses of peppermint tea every day.
- In each cup of peppermint tea, mix in one-eighth of a teaspoon of potassium gluconate.

Make sure you drink the tea consistently as it will help to ease symptoms of nausea and diarrhea. Make sure you use potassium gluconate, not potassium compound. They are different. During this time, there are a few other things you will need to do:

- Only eat oatmeal for your meals three times a day. You can add brown sugar to the oatmeal if you would like and you can also have applesauce.
- During this same time, make sure to switch to chamomile tea enemas instead of coffee enemas. Do this three times a day.

Once you stomach begins to calm down and the diarrhea slows down as well, then you can start adding coffee back to the enemas. Just make sure you mix it with chamomile tea and slowly switch back to water. Start slowly adding juices back as well, but mix then with a couple of ounces of oatmeal gruel. Do not add back foods or medication until the juices can be fully tolerated without oatmeal gruel. When adding foods back, make sure to choose only raw fruits and vegetables because they will be easier to digest.

If diarrhea continues on a small level, grind up charcoal tablets and place them in peppermint tea.

The only time you will need to take further action is if the diarrhea continues for more than three days. Then, you will need to have a stool sample tested to determine what may be going wrong. However, that happens very, very rarely. Most of the time, diarrhea is simply a healing reaction and will go away very quickly.

Depression

What you must remember is that the mind and the body work together. They don't work on their own and each is effected by the other. So, when you experience flare-ups, you may find yourself depressed. This is partly because you may feel as if you are relapsing even if you know that you are dealing with a flare-up. This is also partly because the mind is effected by the body. When the body is detoxifying and changing radically, it will have an impact on the mind.

This depression should only last for the extent of the healing reaction. Additionally, it can be eased with an extra coffee enema.

It is very important to keep in mind that, if you have other serious conditions, then your healing reactions may be different or may be worse. It all depends on your body and how it reacts to being sick. However, as long as you follow proper protocol, then you will be able to get through these healing reactions.

Most of all, when you experience a flare-up, you need to remember these things:

- It is just temporary.
- It means your body is healing.
- You can do things to ease the symptoms.
- Do not stop the therapy.
- Know that the therapy is working.
- The healing reactions are not dangerous.

With those things in mind, you will better be able to get through the flare-ups without worrying that something is wrong and without becoming depressed or assuming you are getting worse instead of better.

Now that we have gone over the bulk of the Gerson Method, the next thing we need to discuss would be pitfalls or mistakes that are commonly made as people attempt to use the treatment to heal themselves.

CHAPTER 10: AVOIDING PITFALLS WHEN USING THE GERSON METHOD

We all make mistakes. It is just a part of being human. Many times, you can simply shrug off a mistake and then move forward past it. The problem on the Gerson Method is that a mistake can set you back quite a great deal in the healing process. To avoid making the mistakes and harming your healing, let's look at the most common pitfalls so that you can avoid them altogether. Obviously, the more you are prepared for mistakes that could happen, the more you will be able to avoid them.

Always Observe the Rules

When you begin Gerson Therapy, you may think at first that the rules are so strict that you may feel like you could never follow them. However, once you get used to the dietary rules, you really can get through it.

No matter what, you cannot break them. There may be a little thought in your head that you can bend them a little here and there – that it won't hurt to have a quick snack – you are very wrong. Even a one bending of the rules can set you back in your healing process extensively. There are a few problems you could run into if you think it is ok to break the rules even a little:

- A little could turn into a lot. Every once in a while can turn into every day.
- Eating something that you shouldn't will immediately put

toxins in your body and will damage your ability to absorb the nutrients you need.
- Your body will become confused because you are sending it the wrong signals.

Honestly, you are going to deal with a couple of things. You will be tempted to eat something you shouldn't just because your body is so used to having the salt and sweets. Additionally, you may have people who are well-meaning albeit dangerous for your progress. They may suggest that the food you are eating isn't good enough or that you really need a big cut of red meat to feel better. When your loved ones are suggesting these things, you may find it very easy to break the rules.

If your loved ones are having trouble understanding your therapy, you may suggest that they learn more about the Gerson Method. You may even recommend that they read this book. Often, they mean well but they don't understand what is going on with your body. When they find out more about the Gerson Method, they will likely stop putting pressure on you to break the rules.

Avoiding Energy Drains

As you start feeling better, you may feel that it is your responsibility to take on more work, especially if your arthritis has kept you from doing things before. However, you must remember that you are still going through the therapy and you are still ill to some extent. Even though you feel much better and you likely have a lot more energy, you are not ready to take on everything right now. Instead, you must continue to get the rest you need. Your body depends on rest to continue healing, so here are some rules that you must keep in mind:

- You should always be in bed no later than 10 pm. This means sleeping, not reading, listening to music, watching television, etc. You need sleep!
- Do not take on extra work, whether that includes around the house or anything else.
- Take an hour long nap in the afternoon as well.

Rest is a must and you need to get plenty of it, even if you are feeling better. So, be sure to continue getting rest no matter what.

Listening to Doctors

To begin with, you are going to need to find an allopathic doctor who respects the Gerson Method and what it can do. A standard medical doctor will be adamantly against you using this therapy. That's because they will almost always recommend using medication. Even when you find an allopathic doctor, though, you could run into problems, so you will have to be very careful.

Often, well-meaning doctors will do blood work, see that certain things are off balance, and then want you to make changes in order to "get those numbers back to normal." The problem with this is that any changes can completely ruin your progress with the method. Additionally, the things that may appear to be out of balance will actually be resolved within just a few days thanks to the Gerson Method.

So, it would most definitely be a pitfall to listen to doctor's recommendations if they suggest you change something about your therapy. Always follow the rules of the protocol so that your healing process can progress as you will want.

Becoming Dejected with Flare-Ups

Flare-ups aren't just common. They are normal and they are a very good thing. They mean your body is healing. If you expect to be the one person who doesn't experience healing reactions, then you will be let down, and you could become so dejected that you want to give up trying. However, since flare-ups are actually a sign that you are healing, you would be giving up on just the right moment when your body is actually making progress.

When you experience healing reactions, then, recognize them as a good thing and be happy. It means your body is taking steps forward.

Using Tap Water

How important is the water, really? You may think and even assume it is completely ok to just use tap water, especially if you don't feel like using the distiller. Sure, just this once I can use tap water, right? This would absolutely be a very big mistake. Tap water is filled with chemicals, including chlorine and fluoride. Both of these are hazardous to your progress with the Gerson Method. Here's a little secret too: even boiling the water will not remove these chemicals from it. So, you have to distill.

What about your bath or shower, you may wonder. Yes, even in the shower, you are exposing yourself to those chemicals and you are keeping your body from healing. For the Gerson Method to work, you have to completely eliminate your exposure to tap water, so you could take a sponge bath with distilled water or use a camp shower filled with distilled water.

Water is extremely important, and that includes what you drink and what you expose your skin to. No matter what, this is a pitfall you absolutely cannot fall for. Use distilled water only if you want the method to actually work.

Trying to Improvise

Everyone knows that the Gerson Method takes a lot of work. You have to:

- Shop for the organic, fresh fruits and vegetables
- Keep those things stored properly
- Remove all chemicals from your home
- Distill your own water
- Prepare your juices and drink them fresh throughout the day
- Prepare fresh meals
- Follow through with the coffee enema protocol
- Clean your house with safe methods

It does take a lot of work, and you may be tempted to cut corners, but a single improvising step can derail your progress completely. Whenever you are tempted to improvise something so that you don't have to take all of the steps, consider your condition. Isn't it truly worth it to go through those steps so that you can live the rest of your life free of arthritis? Of course it is. When you are free from the pain and discomfort, you will certainly be glad you made the decision to follow all of the rules.

Reading the Wrong Information

You know how important it is to read information and study up on the process you will be using, but you have to be very careful, especially if you turn to the Internet to learn more. You will find thousands of different theories and so many contradicting opinions that you will feel completely confused or overwhelmed. It is a good idea to research the Gerson Method, but it is a very bad idea to get your mind muddled by information that will not help you. Additionally, the vast majority of information you could read online will be written by people who aren't experts and don't exactly know what they are talking about.

So, be careful of your sources and study in the correct way.

If you avoid these pitfalls, then you will be able to see the Gerson Method work and you will become healthy. The number one rule you need to always remember is that you have to follow the therapy methods. Don't break the rules and it will work.

CHAPTER 11: YOUR QUESTIONS ANSWERED

Obviously, even after reading everything you have so far, you likely have questions. Of course you do. The Gerson Method is capable of allowing your body to fully heal itself. However, it is completely different from anything you are used to. It can seem quite radical to some people, so questions may abound. In this chapter, we will go over the most common questions you may have and provide you with answers that will help you.

It's completely ok to have questions, so don't feel bad that you need answers.

Can I Use a B-Complex Supplement?

Two different B vitamins are actually used in the Gerson Therapy: B3 and B12. However, other types of vitamins in this same category are actually dangerous and will slow your progress, namely B1 and B6. The B-complex supplements will actually contain everything, including the good and the bad. It simply will not work as an ideal option on the Gerson Therapy. You need to stick with the protocol that has proven to work.

When Can I Have Soy?

Because soy has been touted as healthy for so long and by so many people, you may wonder when you can start having it again.

Unfortunately, you can never have it. In fact, no one should have it. That's because it is toxic and studies have shown that it is toxic even if it is grown organic.

Additionally, soy will block the nutrients you need from absorbing into your system. It is simply unhealthy, so you have to ignore all of the hype out there right now and you need to understand what is actually good and what is actually harmful for you. So, even when you are done with the Gerson Method itself, make sure to never add soy to your diet.

Why Isn't Food Combing a Part of the Therapy?

If you keep up with nutrition news, you have probably seen quite a bit of information about food combining. In the mainstream world, it has become one of the premier ways to eat healthily – or so you have been told. There is a very good reason why the Gerson Method doesn't employ the concept of food combining.

This concept includes high levels of two things you absolutely do not need when you are on the Gerson Method: sodium and animal proteins.

The food combining concept states that you should not mix starch along with fruits, but this is going to happen. That's because fruits and vegetables actually have a certain amount of starch within them. So, the food combining principles simply cannot work with the Gerson Method.

Why Can't I Boil or Steam the Vegetables?

The Gerson Method requires that you cook your vegetables on a very low temperature for an extended period of time. Some people may think this is inconvenient and they may think it would be much simpler to just steam them very quickly. However, exposing vegetables to boiling water or steam (which is hotter than boiling water) will actually change their structure internally. The proteins, enzymes, and nutrients in those fruits and vegetables will be nearly impossible for your body to absorb at this point. Essentially, you will want to allow your food to simmer on very low heat until they are cooked. This will not change their structure and will ensure you get all of their nutritional benefits.

Why Are Potatoes and Tomatoes So Important?

Many of the modern diets or choices in meals recommend avoiding both tomatoes and potatoes. That's because these two are listed as a part of the nightshade family, which is a deadly group of foods. For that reason, you may become very concerned with the fact that the Gerson Method depends strongly on both of them. First of all, they aren't even the main two foods of the therapy! Your main foods will be carrots, apples, and leafy greens.

However, it is important to note that tomatoes and potatoes are nutritious. Potatoes are very easy to digest, which is great for your body, and they have potassium and protein that your body will need to heal itself. Tomatoes are filled with lycopene, which is an antioxidant and has been the subject of many research studies that indicate it is a great boost for your immune system.

Tomatoes and potatoes are not the only healthy vegetables that have been listed as a part of the nightshade family. In fact, the Gerson Method also uses green peppers, and there have been no adverse effects from them. In fact, they are a vital part of healing.

How Long Will Flare-Ups Last?

There is no way to put a number on this. It all has to do with how many toxins are in your body and how much they may have damaged you so far. Some people will only experience flare-ups that last a couple of hours. Others will experience them for more than a day. There is no "normal" here, so be sure to accept the flare-ups as a sign of healing.

How Many Flare-Ups Will I Have?

Again, there is no correct answer to this. Everyone is different. Everyone has been exposed to different levels of toxins and people have different levels of nutritional deficiency. However, there has been enough study into the Gerson Method to somewhat predict when you will actually have healing reactions:

- You will likely have one about one week after beginning the method.

- You will likely have one about six weeks into the treatment.
- You will likely have your most severe flare-ups around three to four months after beginning the treatment.

There is no way to say for certain that this is when you will experience your healing reactions, and you will continue to have them for as long as your body is healing. Don't try to put time frames on your own body because it has to work on its own time.

When I Feel Better, Does This Mean I Am Healed?

You are going to start feeling better very quickly after you begin the treatment – as quickly as a week for many people. That doesn't mean you are healed yet. Instead, it means that your body is starting to heal itself and rid itself of toxins. After about six months, you are probably going to get all of your energy back too. Again, that is because your body is getting stronger.

However, none of this means you are fully healed. Instead, it means you are on the way and you still need to follow the protocol of the Gerson Method. The energy you gain back should be funneled into healing, so don't immediately jump up and start trying to do things. You will be wasting energy that is needed for healing.

Will I Ever Need a Prescription Medication?

The Gerson Method very strongly advises that you should not take prescription medication. These medications have toxic qualities and they don't actually do much to heal you. Instead, they usually just mask conditions and make you worse in other ways.

With that said, there are very rare instances when you may need an antibiotic. If this is the case, then take the medication as recommended and also take the combination of aspirin, vitamin C, and niacin described for Gerson patients. Do not stop your Gerson Therapy during the time you need to take an antibiotic.

Otherwise, any medications prescribed or available over the counter are going to cause side effects, and that tells you immediately that they are toxic for your body.

Will Using Enemas During This Treatment Make Me Dependent on Them?

This is a common question that many people worry over, especially if they have had constipation before. You will not become dependent on enemas. They don't work that way. Once your liver is fully healthy and your intestines are working properly, then everything will do what it should and you won't need enemas anymore.

How Will I Get Protein I Need without Meats?

You have probably been told over and over again that you need animal proteins for a healthy diet. That's because many people are mistaken in what the body actually needs. The types of proteins in animal meat will not work well with your body. Instead, you will get protein from vegetables, and this is the type of protein that can actually be properly digested and absorbed into the body.

Animal proteins can actually feed illness, including tumors, arthritis, and kidney damage. The proteins in fruits and vegetables actually will help heal the body.

You may not realize it, but many vegetables, including carrots, potatoes, and oatmeal are actually very high in proteins.

How Long Will My Therapy Take to Work?

This depends on your illness and how sick you actually are. For most people, it takes about two years for the Gerson Method to fully heal your body. However, that number can vary extensively depending on the situation. This is something you will need to discuss with your specialist.

Are Headaches Normal?

Unfortunately, some people may chalk headaches up to flare-ups, but that is not the case. We discussed the symptoms of healing reactions you should expect with your arthritis treatment already. Headaches are not included in this. Often, a headache may occur when your body is completely overloaded with toxins during the release period. If you experience headaches, then you should add an extra coffee enema each day so that the detoxifying process will work much more quickly. Once the toxins are clear of your body, the headaches should stop.

Now that you have your questions answered, you should feel much more comfortable with every step of the Gerson Method. If you have further questions, you should be able to find the information you need. Just make sure you use only resources that are truly helpful and knowledgeable about the Gerson Method specifically.

You probably deal with a lot of stress. We all do. However, stress is bad for your body and can even slow down the Gerson Method. So, in the next chapter, we are going to talk about ways to reduce stress in your life.

CHAPTER 12: DEALING WITH STRESS

Stress can be so damaging in many different ways. Studies have shown that when you are dealing with chronic stress, you can experience all sorts of side effects, including:

- Weight Gain
- High Blood Pressure
- Irritability
- Headaches
- Fatigue
- Depression
- Lower Immune System

There is even a study out now that shows how chronic stress actually shrinks your brain. Yes, stress is really that bad for you, and it can slow down the Gerson Method too. In fact, this therapy will work the best when you are relaxed and comfortable with your life.

So, in order to use this therapy properly, you should consider ways that you can relax and remove stress from your life.

Here are some options you could consider.

Meditation

Meditation has long been used as a de-stressing method because it works to help clear your brain. When you meditate, you are actually choosing to clear your mind and making the decision to allow yourself to relax. There are different ways you can meditate, but here are some things to keep in mind:

- Find a quiet place where you can relax. That could be in a room, a closet, or even in the woods. You just need to get away from distractions.
- Make sure you are completely comfortable. That means you feel comfortable in your clothing, the room is the right temperature, and nothing painful is distracting. Many people choose to sit on blankets or cushions to ensure their comfort.
- Set apart about a 30 minutes to an hour for meditation. Do not just to force time into your day to meditate. If you do this, then you will actually be thinking about everything you need to do when you are supposed to be relaxing your mind.

To meditate, go to your quiet, comfortable spot. Then, be in the moment. That means being aware of yourself completely and totally. Focus on your breathing. Imagine the air coming in and out of your lungs. Be aware of every part of you, from your hair to your toes. Don't let your mind think of anything else but yourself in the present.

When you do this, you will clear your mind of every other thought and you will focus on awareness. This will allow you to relax and take some time away from stress. It can work wonders for relaxing through the rest of the day too.

Visualization

You can actually use visualization in conjunction with meditation because it will allow you to take your relaxation technique a step further. So, try this the next time you spend an hour or so meditating:

- As you reach your meditative state, you are going to actually start visualizing something.
- Close your eyes and see something in your mind. The image you see should be what you will look and feel like when you are well from your arthritis. Really focus on this image. Think of it like a painting that you paint each stroke carefully. Once

you have that painting in your mind, then move on to the next step.
- With the painting clear and before you, visualize stepping into it. The painting will become real and you will be surrounded by it. See it, feel it, smell it, hear it – use all of your senses to see that perfect image of you without stress and without arthritis.
- Now, step back out of that painting and look at the steps it took for you to get to that perfect image. When you can imagine the steps, then you will see exactly what you need to do in order to get here.

As you come out of the meditative state, you will be more relaxed in knowing that you have something to work toward – something that can be very real for you. Not only will this help you relax, but also it will help you to have the motivation you need so that you can move forward with the Gerson Method.

Take Some Time for Yourself

The most important thing you need to keep in mind when you work on removing stress from your life is that you do need to take some time for yourself. Just get away from any responsibilities and from doing things for other people. Each day, set aside that time to meditate, read, listen to music, work on a hobby, or do anything that just works as "me" time.

Work on Gratitude

When you live a life of gratitude, you will find that there is no room for stress and negativity in your life. So, work on becoming more grateful. There are several ways you could do this:

- Every morning, spend a few moments thinking of at least five things you are grateful for.
- Create a gratitude journal. Each day, you can write things down that you are grateful for.

- Write gratitude notes. This is especially helpful for showing gratitude toward other people. There is nothing wrong with saying thank you, and it will make you feel better.

The Gerson Method is successful, but it will work more quickly and efficiently when you eliminate stress from your life, so work on this and ensure that your therapy is working as well as possible.

Now that we have discussed the Gerson Method and how you can use it, we can move on to focusing on what will come after the treatment itself. That's what we will discuss in the next chapter.

CHAPTER 13: WHAT TO EXPECT AFTER THE GERSON METHOD

Once you have completed the Gerson Therapy, you will need to come off of it in the right way. It's not as simple as just going back to what you were eating. That would be detrimental to your health. So, you need to understand what you will need to do in order to continue living the rest of your life healthily once you are down with the Gerson Method.

The number one rule you should remember is that it is better to stay on the method longer instead of coming off of it too soon. There is no harm that can come from staying on the therapy longer, but there is great harm in taking yourself off of it too soon.

To stop your therapy, you will need to follow these steps:

- This will be a gradual process. Do not just try to stop on one day.
- Slowly reduce your coffee enemas until you are using them twice a week.
- Slowly cut down your juices to five or six a day.

Once you get to this point, you should consider sticking with that protocol for the rest of your life. It will allow you to remain very healthy from now on.

Beyond that, there are some things we need to discuss about how you can make wise choices about how you live your life and what you eat.

Maintenance

As you come off of your Gerson Method, you will actually go back to living a normal life, with some rules in place. You still need to make wise decisions about what you eat, such as you do need to avoid animal proteins, but you can follow a looser diet now. This will allow you to go to events like banquets, wedding receptions, etc. and find things to eat. However, during the maintenance phase of your life, you will need to follow a few rules as well:

- If you do "binge" and allow yourself to eat things that aren't necessarily considered healthy, you will need to do a couple of things in the next few days to ensure your body stays healthy.
- After one of these events, go back to doing daily coffee enemas.
- After these events, take a digestive enzyme for two or three days until anything toxic has passed from your system.

You should also consider doing the full Gerson Method program a couple of times a year. That way, you will completely flush your body and this will help your system keep the health it gained while you were doing the method in the first place. The best way to do this is to choose two weeks a year, far apart from each other of course, and use the Gerson Method once again for each of those weeks.

Making Smart Choices

Even though you will be done with the Gerson Method, there are still things you need to do in order to make smart choices. You simply would be making a very big mistake if you start feeding your body toxins. Here are a few things to keep in mind:

- You should never go back to eating fast foods. They are filled with toxins, especially sodium.
- You should never start eating junk foods as they are filled with additives as well.
- You should continue buying only organic foods and

vegetables. Non-organic foods are filled with pesticides and other chemicals.
- Continue eating "protective" foods. These are organic fruits and vegetables that will specifically help your body maintain its health.
- If you really want to drink alcohol, it needs to be done very rarely and very carefully. Make sure any alcohol you choose has to be organic.

It will be very important that you approach your life after the Gerson Method very carefully. That's because you don't want to undo everything good you have done for your body while you were on the therapy. As long as you approach your removal of the therapy very slowly and you make smart choices with your foods, then you will be able to maintain a healthy life despite no longer being on the therapy itself.

CHAPTER 14: FURTHER RESOURCES

Of course, it is always a good idea to learn more whenever you can. The more you can research and use the Gerson Method, the better off you will be. It is important to avoid any of the confusing and overwhelming information you could run into, so instead of searching out information all on your own, look into these resources.

Begin by going to the Gerson Institute webpage, where you will find a variety of different resources that can help you learn more. It's available at www.gerson.org. Not only will you find details on Gerson Therapy, but also you will find recipes and even details on what types of cleaning and hygiene products you can use.

When you begin looking for equipment to buy for your kitchen, this buying guide can be helpful. It goes over different juicers you could purchase. Look up the buying guide at www.foodmatters.tv/juicer-buying-guide

This buying guide has different types of coffee, but you can look at the organic section to consider your options. Look it up at www.consumerreports.org/cro/coffee/buying-guide.htm.

When you need to purchase supplies and supplements, there are different places you can shop, including:

- The Key Company, www.thekeycompanyusa.com
- Stat MX, www.statmx.com
- Ishi Medical Equipment, www.ishimedical.com
- Healing Naturally Limited, www.healingnaturally.co.uk
- Nutricology, www.nutricology.com

- Biogenesis Anti-Aging, www.biogenesis-antiaging.com

These companies will help you get different supplies and medications you will need for your Gerson Therapy.

If you would like to read the books written by Charlotte and Max Gerson, here is a listing of them:

- The Gerson Therapy: The Proven Nutritional Program for Cancer and Other Illnesses by Charlotte Gerson and Morton Walker
- Healing the Gerson Way by Charlotte Gerson
- Defeating Obesity, Diabetes, and High Blood Pressure, by Charlotte Gerson
- A Cancer Therapy: Results of Fifty Cases and the Cure of Advanced Cancer by Diet Therapy by Max Gerson

Of course, the more you read, the more you can fully understand how Gerson Therapy can help you.

CONCLUSION

As you can see, the Gerson Method has shown to be very effective, and it doesn't just help people with cancer. This therapy has proven time and again that it can heal a variety of different conditions, and that includes arthritis.

Right now, you are dealing with a condition, and you have probably been told there is no cure. That's not the case, no matter what type of arthritis you may have. The condition is caused by two main things: lack of nutrients that your body needs and a buildup of toxicity within your liver and the rest of your body. Those two things together make you sick, and the only way to become well is to correct them.

The most important thing to remember is that your body is fully capable of healing itself. It can get well. All you need to do is give it the tools it requires. Once you remove all of the toxins from your body and you take them out of your environment, your body can begin healing itself. Then, when you give it the nutrients it needs, your body will get well.

It's amazing what the human body is capable of when it is allowed to do what it does best: stay healthy.

And, the big news is that it has nothing to do with typical medications. Those medications just cover up illness and don't make you better. They have so many side effects that they are likely to make you worse. They aren't the answer. Your body is the answer and when you use the Gerson Method, you will find that it can truly heal itself.

Throughout this book, we have discussed everything you need to know in order to live a healthy life, and the best part is, the therapy won't just heal your arthritis. It will heal everything else wrong with your body as well.

So, instead of spending another day sick, in pain, and uncomfortable, it is time to do something different. Start the Gerson Method now and realize you can live a fully healthy life.

David Robin

www.ingramcontent.com/pod-product-compliance
Lightning Source LLC
Chambersburg PA
CBHW070806220526
45466CB00002B/567